Check-up on it!

Breast Cancer:
365 days to track your breast health

Journal

This Journal belongs to:

13ᵀᴴ & JOAN

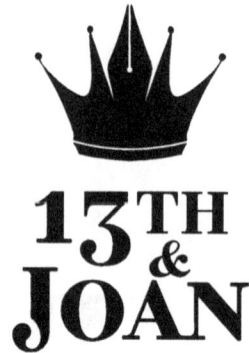

For permission requests, write to the publisher, addressed "Attention: Permissions Coordinator," 205 N. Michigan Avenue, Suite #810, Chicago, IL 60601. 13th & Joan books may be purchased for educational, business or sales promotional use. For information, please email the Sales Department at sales@13thandjoan.com.

Printed in the U. S. A.

First Printing, May 2024

Library of Congress Cataloging-in-Publication Data has been applied for.

ISBN: 978-1-961863-26-2

This one is for you, you, my number one.....

Dedication and Acknowledgements

THIS IS FOR every breast cancer survivor, the families, and those who did not win the individual war but helped with advancements in the medical field to help save others' lives. I designed this journal for me, a Black woman, who is overlooked and whose thoughts on my health are undervalued. I dedicate this journal to every person who has felt invisible during their health journey. I see you.

Thank you to my family, friends, and therapist who gave me feedback, encouragement, and held me accountable to ensure this journal made it to the physical form and did not just remain in my mind. Thank you for reading, reviewing, and editing my countless text messages and emails. You are the real MVPs!

I go for mine, I gots to shine.....

Endorsements

"This is wonderful and heartfelt. I had a few extra emotions reading this, as I have lost a family member to breast cancer. I appreciate the "how-to." As Americans, a woman's body is taught to be shameful to many. This just reiterates that doing an exam is for your health, nothing to be ashamed of, and what to pay attention to if something seems different. Also, I appreciate the emotion wheel. I would have never thought of having a ready-made description area to enter and reflect on your feelings or how this could really benefit a person until I sat with how people feel when receiving a scary diagnosis. I am proud of you! This is going to help many, many people. *I look forward to the publication.*"

– Corinne Brant,
Personal Fitness Instructor

"In the intimate embrace of your own strength and vulnerability, this journal becomes a sacred journey–a testament to the resilience within. With each stroke of the pen, you paint a masterpiece of self-care and self-discovery, as you traverse the peaks and valleys of life, armed with love, knowledge, and a woman of an indomitable spirit. I am eager to share this simple yet detailed journal with those that I encounter in the hopes it provides a slight ease of mental anguish they may experience during a pivotal time in their life."

– Kenya Turner Washington,
Clinical Social Worker/Therapist
LCSW of Kenya's Way (kenyasway.org)

"BRAVO! 💗 ✨ #Simply Amazing!!!!! Well worth the read and should be placed in all health centers around the world. As a woman, I thank you!!!!!!!!!"

– TaMonica S.,
Medical Assistant & Health Center Support Reception

Contents

The reason why you found this journal

FEBRUARY 2021, ONE year into the pandemic. It was just an ordinary day when I interrupted my mom's work day to talk to me while I drove to my doctor's appointment. I took the elevator to the right to the second floor. I rushed my mom off the phone as I entered the suite. I checked in at the counter, then finished and returned my paperwork. I watched HGTV that was playing on TV as the sun shined through the window, creating the deception of warmth on what was a chilly day. It seemed to take longer than usual to be seen, but I was in no rush to return to the office. The nurse came out and started to stutter my name, Martricia, Martrika. I corrected her with a nice tone. *"Yes, Martrica, Mar-tree-sa. Everyone always mispronounces my name."* I placed my items in the chair to the left to step on the scale. I cringed at the number and hurriedly stepped off. I gathered my things to have a seat for my blood pressure. I sat looking at all the pictures of the babies that the doctor delivered. I started taking a slightly deeper breath because the compression was super tight. The nurse broke my breathing concentration and told me my numbers were good and to follow her. I got up and followed her to the last room on the left at the end of the hall. None of that meant much at the time, but the foreshadowing was eerie.

I walked in and followed the normal protocol. I took off each piece of clothing and wrapped my undergarments inside of my clothes. I casually scrolled through social media. I waited and waited. I heard the nurse and doctor fiddling with the door, so I began to shuffle like a child who is doing something they have no business doing. I hurried to place my phone on top of my clothes. I tried to stay focused as she asked me questions about my health and then the exam began. Right arm up, chit chat, chit chat, right arm down. Left arm up and I am exposed. The cold made me shiver. Three finger tips made circles with different pressure levels. A pause and then the words you never want to hear. *"I think I found something. May I have your hand?"* All I can hear is the crinkling of the white paper sheets I am laying on as she takes my hand and places it on the inside of my left breast. It's small, but it is something. I mustered up the nerve and said, *"Yes, I feel it."* I was flooded with emotion as my doctor told me that it could be nothing, but she wanted to send me to get a mammogram at the tender age of 34–just a few months shy of my 35th birthday. In just a few days ,the mammogram was completed and the results were in......negative. *"Thank goodness, life can proceed as normal."* Well, at least that's what I thought.

Fast forward to September 2021, at home doing a self breast exam laying in the center of the primary bedroom's bed. The TV played in the background and the AC kicked on to cool the house on that hot Oklahoma evening. Suddenly, I felt the same coldness from March while circling my breast, the right breast now. I thought I felt something. I was nervous! I had my roommate confirm. They can feel it too. My thoughts were roaming from one end of the universe to the other. I did my best to convince myself that I was imagining things and was not feeling a pea- sized unidentified object in my body! I did what I do best when I have a bad day: I went to sleep to clear my thoughts before working on next steps. In the middle of the night, I started crafting a message to my doctor via MyChart. I was blinded by a stream of tears that created a small puddle on my pillow. I stopped and put my phone up and attempted to get more rest.

I rose to the sunniest day and a blue sky, but it was all the reverse reflection of my emotions. I put on a happy and brave face in lieu of the blue sadness of worry in mind. I made it to the office early to complete my email, which detailed everything I could think of with the help of Google. The doctor's office sent me an email and scheduled my appointment within a week. The doctor confirmed that she felt something and ordered a mammogram and ultrasound. This time around, it took a week or so to get the tests completed. I heard the chime of the incoming email on my phone. I opened the email and of course, I had to sign in to the MyChart website. I couldn't remember one of the million passwords I used on a regular basis. News of my health was held hostage by a password. After a couple failed password attempts, I finally succeeded. I clicked on the message box and took a deep breath. The following were my results and subsequent conversation with the doctor's office.

Narrative

BILATERAL DIGITAL DIAGNOSTIC MAMMOGRAM 3D/2D AND TARGETED RIGHT ULTRASOUND: 9/28/2021

HISTORY: Diffuse right breast pain within the upper inner quadrant. Palpable lump within the right breast at the 3 o'clock position.

COMPARISON: No prior exams were available for comparison.

TECHNIQUE: 3D tomographic images were obtained in multiple projections of both breasts.

BREAST COMPOSITION: The breasts are heterogeneously dense, which may obscure small masses (ACR category c).

FINDINGS: No significant masses, calcifications, or other findings are seen in either breast mammographically. No significant abnormalities were seen sonographically in the right breast.

IMPRESSION: ACR BI-RADS CATEGORY 1: NEGATIVE, ULTRASOUND ACR BI-RADS CATEGORY 1: NEGATIVE

There is no abnormality seen in the right breast to correspond with the diffuse pain in the upper inner quadrant. Patient was provided with information about breast pain and management options.

There is no abnormality seen in the right breast to correspond with the palpable abnormality at 3 o'clock. Follow-up clinical breast examination is recommended in three months.

There is no mammographic or sonographic evidence of malignancy. Begin routine annual screening at age 40.

Given increased breast density and/or intermediate risk for developing breast cancer, supplemental screening with automated whole breast ultrasound is recommended in this patient.

The patient was notified of the results.

IN A BLINK of an eye, I time traveled back to high school sitting in Intro to Spanish. I was striving to read this foreign language of doctor jargon and allow my brain to process syllable by syllable, word by word, but I was not grasping what it meant. The information left my mind on the darkest country road, miles away from civilization, and nobody heard my cries. I was lost, my tank was empty but filled with the unknown regarding my health. Maybe I needed to cry at the moment, maybe I needed to find some resolve, or just maybe a lot of both! I took the third option and worked to get some answers to my confusion. I was determined to fix the lack of communication and the convoluted doctor talk. I called but could not reach anyone at the doctor's office. So, I whipped out my computer, determined to get the answers to stop my mind from pacing back and forth on that dark country road.

I completed my mammogram and was unable to find anything. However, I am concerned with the test details written up. I am requesting clarity.

In the details it stated that they did not have anything to compare this mammogram to a previous one. However, I completed a mammogram back in March 2021 which they could have compared and I assume they did not. Can they compare the mammogram from March 2021 to the one from yesterday?

- *The tech asked if I drank caffeine and I told her no, not really, that I drink water, juice, and Italian soda sometimes. At the end of the visit, she provided me with a sheet about pain management and caffeine.*
- *I was not informed that I would need a three-month follow-up. The tech advised me to check monthly to verify what I am feeling and if it grows while I described the 5 cm lump to her. I would like a three-month follow-up but with another facility.*
- *I was not told the following...Given increased breast density and/or intermediate risk for developing breast cancer, supplemental screening with automated whole breast ultrasound is recommended in this patient. If this is the case, why is it recommended to start routine mammograms at 40? Please advise.*

I knew I would get answers! I made it clear where my confusion lied. As I continued with my day, I got another ping.

They typically use old mammograms to compare. It appears that you have some breast density and that is the reason for the breast ultrasound. I will get that ordered for you. The recommendation is that we get those results and then will proceed after we get those results back. That will tell us what the next steps should be.

Well, that was not what I was expecting. Nothing had really been addressed. My frustrations were growing, and I was no closer to any answers. I was more confused by the contradicting reply. Maybe there was some kind of mix-up or they did not go back and read my previous history charts. *"Let's try this again,"* I thought. I sent another email and made a few call-outs!

Thank you, it was listed in my testing results and I was a little confused about what they listed about the breast density. I thought the results were sent to you and me at the same time. I will wait for your review of the test results and recommendation.

I did not receive any additional communication via MyChart. I called to follow up and within the next day or so, I received a letter in the mail advising me to have an automated breast ultrasound (ABS) partnered with a phone call from the doctor's office. I spoke to the nurse and she educated me on the ABS procedure and how some insurance companies do not cover the cost, which could be up to $1,500. It was recommended I have the test every six months, which again contradicted the recommendation in my results to begin routine annual screening at age 40.

A while passed and my annual check-up came. I realized that I never had my ABS conducted. My doctor ordered the ABS, which was partially covered by my insurance and ended up costing $500 out of pocket. It was worth every penny when the results came back negative.

These interactions put my semi-control freak nature in a frenzy, and I had no place to home it. Where could I place my emotions, my concerns, my proactiveness, my unknowns, my control, and more? I was back down the dark country road, but I spotted a proverbial bright blinking porch light in the distance. I hunted down the light and was able to find a home for my control, concern, emotions, nerves, proactiveness, and more. That light led me home to my own voice in my medical journey. I decided to be my own health advocate and take control of my health, even though my results were still negative. I was unsuccessful in finding a journal that would cover every aspect of breast health, which resulted in the birth of this breast health journal. During my breast health journey, I worked over the next year or more to develop this journal as a companion down the dark and lonely road.

It does not matter if you are completely "healthy," if you have a health scare, or are in the midst of your health storm. We all have a sense of needing and wanting to be in control, especially when we feel we do not have any. Take back your control. You can do that as long as you are being an advocate for you, your health, and your well-being. You will always be doing the right thing when it comes to your health. My hope for you is to use this journal to know that you are not alone, you have a place in your health journey, and you cannot offend anyone by asking questions about your body. Cultural experiences are important, so find someone who can educate you the way you need them to. Use this journal to hunt down your light and find home in your voice. Allow it to shield and comfort you during your time of being OK, going forward through darkness, or working through the unknown.

A Call to Live

Why should you take breast cancer seriously at any age and regardless of your ethnicity?

Because your individualism and your life matter, therefore you matter.

INCIDENCE RATES OF breast cancer vary among different ethnic groups. Here are some general trends in the United States based on Susan B. Komen statics:

- Non-Hispanic white women have the highest incidence rates of breast cancer.
- African American women have slightly lower incidence rates compared to non-Hispanic white women, but they have a higher mortality rate and are more likely to be diagnosed at a later stage.
- Hispanic women have lower incidence rates compared to non-Hispanic white and African American women.
- Asian/Pacific Islander women have the lowest incidence rates among all ethnic groups.
- American Indian/Alaska Native women have lower incidence rates compared to non-Hispanic white women.

It's important to note that these statements are based on general trends. Individual experiences may vary.

The U.S. is not alone in the cancer battle. Out of 184 countries, breast cancer was the common diagnosis for women in 140 countries, according to the Breast Cancer Research Foundation.

Breast cancer mortality rates can also vary among different ethnic groups. African American women tend to have higher mortality rates compared to women of other ethnicities. Factors contributing to this disparity include differences in healthcare access, socioeconomic status, tumor characteristics, and genetic factors.

According to the Centers for Disease Control and Prevention (CDC), genetic factors can play a role in cancer. Specific gene mutations can increase the risk of developing breast cancer. For example, certain BRCA1 and BRCA2 gene mutations are more prevalent among women of Ashkenazi Jewish descent.

These mutations are associated with a higher risk of developing breast and ovarian cancers. Genetic testing and counseling can help identify individuals who may be at higher risk.

Importance of self-breast exams

Self-breast exams are a way for women to become familiar with the normal look and feel of their breasts so they can detect any changes or abnormalities. While self-breast exams are not a substitute for regular mammograms or clinical breast exams, they can serve as an early detection tool. Women should consult with their healthcare providers to understand the appropriate frequency and technique for self-breast exams.

Screening guidelines

Regular mammograms and clinical breast exams are important for breast cancer screening. Guidelines may vary depending on age, family history, and individual risk factors. In the United States, general recommendations include mammograms starting at age 40 or earlier for higher-risk individuals, clinical breast exams every 1-3 years for women in their 20s and 30s, and annually for women 40 and older.

Importance of early detection

Early detection of breast cancer is crucial for better treatment outcomes. Regular screenings, including mammograms and clinical breast exams along with self-breast exams, can help identify breast abnormalities at an early stage when treatment options are more effective.

It's important to remember that breast cancer risk and experiences can vary widely among individuals. Healthcare professionals should be consulted for personalized advice on screening and prevention strategies based on individual risk factors.

I know this is a lot to take in and is sobering, however, we need to wrap ourselves in knowledge and be proactive. Most of us treat and maintain our vehicles better than our bodies. Getting the oil change and tire rotation every six months, filling up the tank, washing the vehicle weekly or bi-weekly, and more! Be just as proactive in your health. These facts and this journal are not just a call to action or a walk-up call. Look at it as aiding in saving your own life because you took action and did not wait until you randomly noticed a change in your body. Putting a routine in place and becoming a self-advocate can help you discover changes sooner than later.

Keep on using me, until you use me up!

How to use this journal

WHEN IT COMES to breast cancer prevention and early detection, keeping a breast health journal can be a powerful tool. By recording any changes or abnormalities in your breasts, you can track any potential warning signs and take action early on.

In addition to tracking physical changes, it's also important to note any lifestyle factors that could impact breast health, such as alcohol consumption, smoking, or exposure to environmental toxins.

By keeping a detailed breast health journal, you can take an active role in your breast health and catch any potential issues early on. Remember to always consult with your healthcare provider if you have any concerns or notice any changes in your breasts.

You will manage your medical records in the Health Records section. This is an easy way to keep track of all of the doctors and medical procedures. This section allows your loved ones to be informed of details during a medical emergency. If you receive regular mammograms or other breast screenings, make a note of the date and results. This will help you keep track of any changes over time and ensure you're staying up-to-date on your screenings.

Whether you have medical insurance or not, you will accrue medical expenses. Use the Check up on your Expenses section to keep track of your running medical expenses.

Get to Know your Breast section is designed to build a monthly routine. Here you will get to know your breast on an intimate level and will be able to recognize any changes in your breast. Use the At-Home Breast Exam to guide you in facilitating an at-home exam and What to look for when checking your breast will show you how to identify concerns. First, start by noting the date of your menstrual cycle, as hormonal changes can affect breast tissue. Then, perform a self-breast exam and record any lumps, bumps, or changes in texture or appearance. It's also important to note any pain, tenderness, or discharge.

The following sections were created to help you along the journey if you have an abnormality: Get your questions answered by your doctor, Know Your Results, Check in: Doctor's appointment, Chemo, Radiation, Surgery appointment, daily routine. These sections will allow you to acknowledge your feelings during, before, and after your appointments, as well as help you prepare for your doctor's appointment and to actively participate in your health.

Lastly, if you have more thoughts or additional notes, use the Notes section.

The correct way to check your breast health: Check 1, Check 2, Check 3, Check 4

How to perform a breast exam at home

IT IS IMPORTANT to regularly perform breast exams at home as a way to detect changes and abnormalities that may be early signs of breast cancer. Early detection is vital for improving treatment outcomes and survival rates.

Instructions for performing a breast exam:

- **Step 1:** Stand in front of a mirror with your arms by your sides. Look for any changes in the size, shape, or appearance of your breasts, such as swelling, dimpling, or redness.
- **Step 2:** Raise your arms above your head and look for the same changes.
- **Step 3:** Lie down on a flat surface with a pillow under one shoulder. Using the pads of your fingers, press down on your breast in a circular motion, starting at the outer edges and moving inward. Make sure to cover the entire breast, including the armpit area.
- **Step 4:** Repeat the exam on the other breast.
- **Step 5:** Feel for any lumps or abnormalities.

When to consult a healthcare provider:
If you notice any changes or abnormalities during your breast exam, it's important to bring them to the attention of your healthcare provider.

It's also a good idea to schedule regular check-ups with your healthcare provider, even if you don't notice any changes.

Being proactive in your breast health by performing regular at-home exams and staying up-to-date with your healthcare provider.

The correct way to check your breast health:
Check 1, Check 2, Check 3, Check 4

At Home Breast Exam

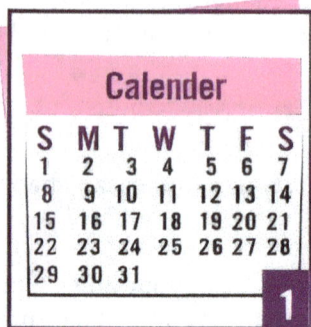

**Self check
once a month**

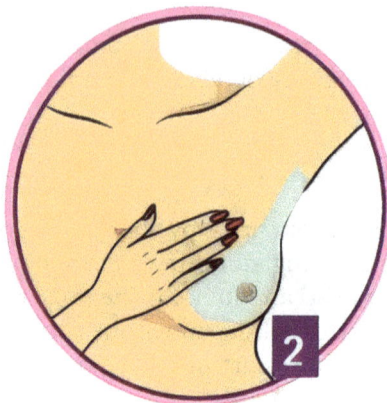

**Examine entire breast
and armpit area**

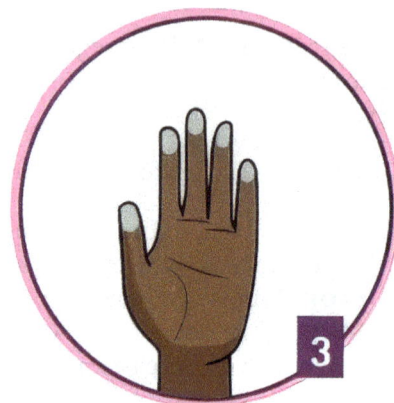

**Gently use the pads
of the fingertips**

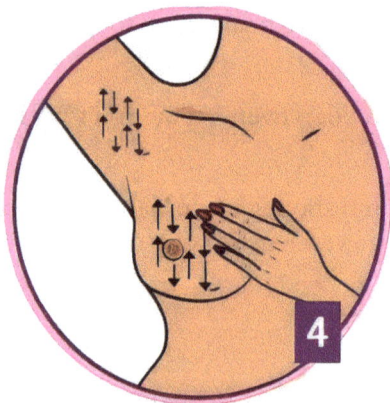

Top and bottom

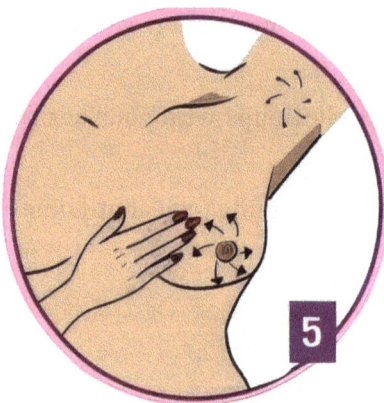

Semi-circles

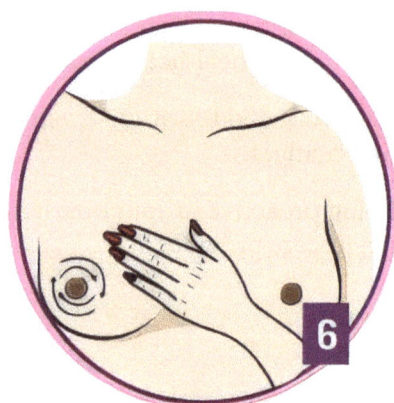

Circles

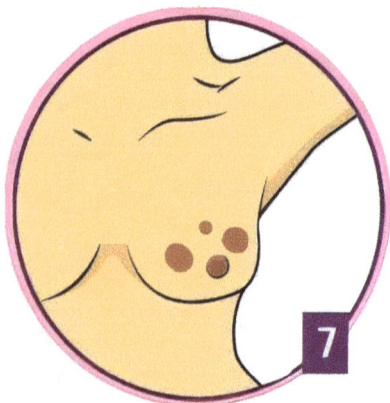

**Look in the mirror
for visual lumps**

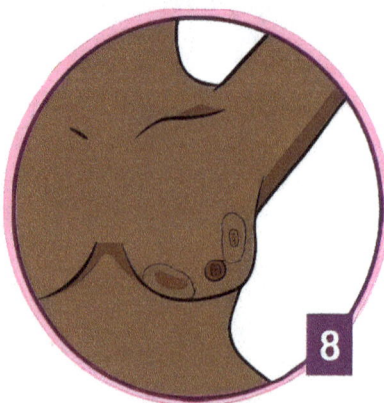

**...skin and texture
changes...**

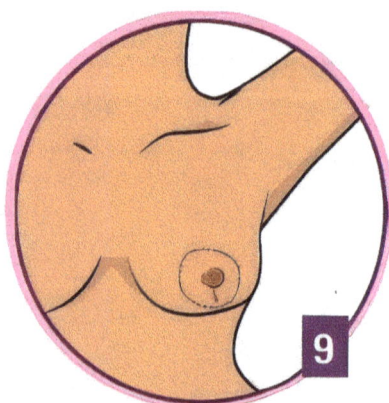

**...changes in nipple shape
or abnormal discharge**

10

The correct way to check your breast health: Check 1, Check 2, Check 3, Check 4

Are you showing signs of these common symptoms of suspected breast cancer?

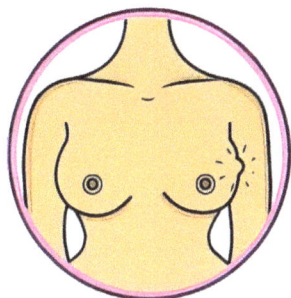

Lumps

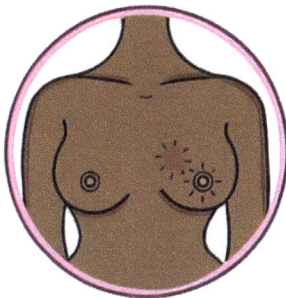

Breast or nipple pain

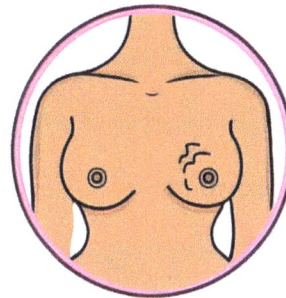

Changes to skin texture

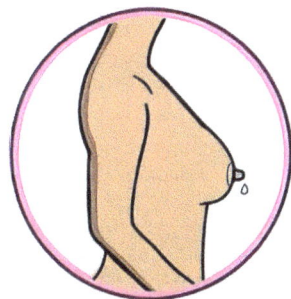

Nipple discharge

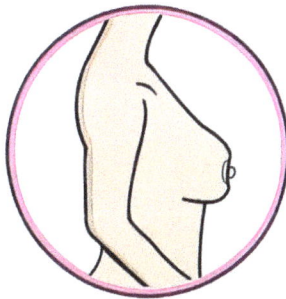

Nipple retraction or inversion

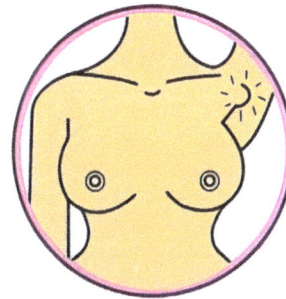

Lymph node changes Lump in armpit

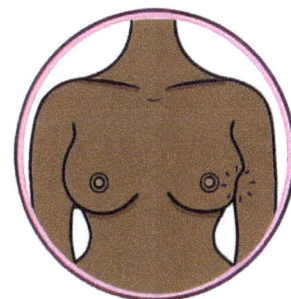

Dimpling

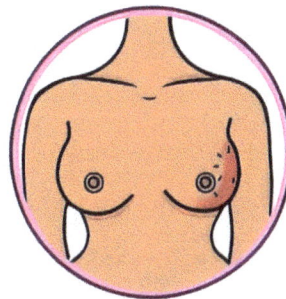

Redness

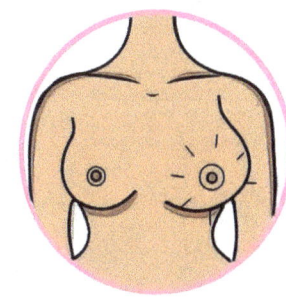

Swelling

Keeping up with your health records

Your Info

Name:

Phone No.:

Emergency Contact:

Phone No.:

Insurance

Provider:

Policy number:

Doctors

Primary doctor:

Specialist's Name & Specialty:

Primary's Phone No.:

Specialist's Phone No.:

Known Conditions, Allergies, & Medications

Condition	Description	Medication

Additional Doctors

Primary doctor:	*Primary's Phone No.:*
Specialist's Name & Specialty:	*Specialist's Phone No.:*
Specialist's Name & Specialty:	*Specialist's Phone No.:*
Specialist's Name & Specialty:	*Specialist's Phone No.:*
Specialist's Name & Specialty:	*Specialist's Phone No.:*

Known Conditions, Allergies, & Medications

Condition	Description	Medication

Keeping up with your health records

Your Info

Name:

Emergency
Contact:

Phone No.:

Phone No.:

Insurance

Provider:

Policy
number:

Doctors

Primary
doctor:

Primary's
Phone No.:

Specialist's Name
& Specialty:

Specialist's
Phone No.:

Known Conditions, Allergies, & Medications

Condition	Description	Medication

Additional Doctors

Primary doctor:	*Primary's Phone No.:*
Specialist's Name & Specialty:	*Specialist's Phone No.:*
Specialist's Name & Specialty:	*Specialist's Phone No.:*
Specialist's Name & Specialty:	*Specialist's Phone No.:*
Specialist's Name & Specialty:	*Specialist's Phone No.:*

Known Conditions, Allergies, & Medications

Condition	Description	Medication

Keep up with your health records

Surgeries		
Date	**Description**	**Facility**

Keep up with your health records

Surgeries		
Date	**Description**	**Facility**

Keep up with your health records

Surgeries		
Date	**Description**	**Facility**

Keep up with your health records

Surgeries		
Date	**Description**	**Facility**

Keep up with your expenses

Date	Description	Due Date	Amount	Paid

Keep up with your expenses

Date	Description	Due Date	Amount	Paid

Keep up with your expenses

Date	Description	Due Date	Amount	Paid

Keep up with your expenses

Date	Description	Due Date	Amount	Paid

Keep up with your expenses

Date	Description	Due Date	Amount	Paid

Keep up with your expenses

Date	Description	Due Date	Amount	Paid

Keep up with your expenses

Date	Description	Due Date	Amount	Paid

Keep up with your expenses

Date	Description	Due Date	Amount	Paid

Keep up with your expenses

Date	Description	Due Date	Amount	Paid

Keep up with your expenses

Date	Description	Due Date	Amount	Paid

Keep up with your expenses

Date	Description	Due Date	Amount	Paid

Keep up with your expenses

Date	Description	Due Date	Amount	Paid

Keep up with your expenses

Date	Description	Due Date	Amount	Paid

Keep up with your expenses

Date	Description	Due Date	Amount	Paid

Keep up with your expenses

Date	Description	Due Date	Amount	Paid

Keep up with your expenses

Date	Description	Due Date	Amount	Paid

Keep up with your expenses

Date	Description	Due Date	Amount	Paid

Keep up with your expenses

Date	Description	Due Date	Amount	Paid

Keep up with your expenses

Date	Description	Due Date	Amount	Paid

Keep up with your expenses

Date	Description	Due Date	Amount	Paid

Get your questions answered by your doctor

TOP PRIORITIES

1	
2	
3	

DATE	QUESTIONS FOR DR.	ANSWERS/NOTES

Get your questions answered by your doctor

TOP PRIORITIES

1	
2	
3	

DATE	QUESTIONS FOR DR.	ANSWERS/NOTES

Get your questions answered by your doctor

TOP PRIORITIES

1	
2	
3	

DATE	QUESTIONS FOR DR.	ANSWERS/NOTES

Get your questions answered by your doctor

TOP PRIORITIES

1	
2	
3	

DATE	QUESTIONS FOR DR.	ANSWERS/NOTES

Get your questions answered by your doctor

TOP PRIORITIES

1	
2	
3	

DATE	QUESTIONS FOR DR.	ANSWERS/NOTES

Know your results

DATE	TEST/VISIT	RESULTS

Hopes

SELF-CARE

Know your results

DATE	TEST/VISIT	RESULTS

Hopes

SELF-CARE

Know your results

DATE	TEST/VISIT	RESULTS

Hopes

SELF-CARE

Know your results

DATE	TEST/VISIT	RESULTS

Hopes

SELF-CARE

Know your results

DATE	TEST/VISIT	RESULTS

Hopes

SELF-CARE

Know your results

DATE	TEST/VISIT	RESULTS

Hopes

SELF-CARE

Know your results

DATE	TEST/VISIT	RESULTS

Hopes

SELF-CARE

Know your results

DATE	TEST/VISIT	RESULTS

Hopes

SELF-CARE

Get to know your breasts

DATE _____   TIME _____

Left	Right
Do you notice any changes?	Do you notice any changes?

Overall Breast Health

	Yes	No	If yes, what is different?
Bulging of skin	☐	☐	
Color	☐	☐	
Dimpling	☐	☐	
Puckering	☐	☐	
Shape	☐	☐	
Size	☐	☐	
Swelling	☐	☐	
Pain	☐	☐	1 2 3 4 5 6 7 8 9 10
Soreness	☐	☐	1 2 3 4 5 6 7 8 9 10

	Yes	No	If yes, what is different?
Bulging of skin	☐	☐	
Color	☐	☐	
Dimpling	☐	☐	
Puckering	☐	☐	
Shape	☐	☐	
Size	☐	☐	
Swelling	☐	☐	
Pain	☐	☐	1 2 3 4 5 6 7 8 9 10
Soreness	☐	☐	1 2 3 4 5 6 7 8 9 10

Nipple

Position	☐	☐
Ex: position change: Inward instead of pushing outward		
Redness	☐	☐
Ex: Position change: Inward instead of pushing outward		
Fluid	☐	☐
Ex: blood, milky, yellow fluid, or watery		

Position	☐	☐
Ex: position change: Inward instead of pushing outward		
Redness	☐	☐
Ex: Position change: Inward instead of pushing outward		
Fluid	☐	☐
Ex: blood, milky, yellow fluid, or watery		

Lump

Bulging of skin	☐	☐
Color	☐	☐
Dimpling	☐	☐

Bulging of skin	☐	☐
Color	☐	☐
Dimpling	☐	☐

Next steps: Notified Dr. ☐   Dr's Appointment ☐

Label Lump, pain, and/or create your own label

USE L = LUMP   **USE P = PAIN**

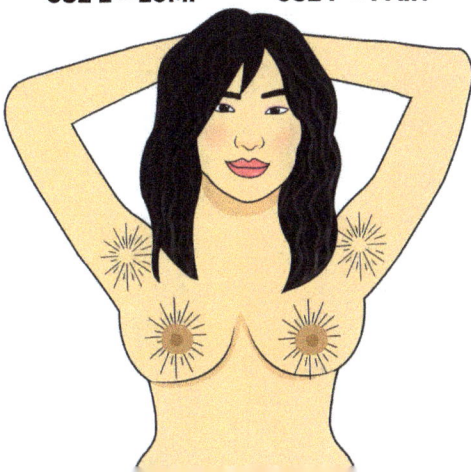

HAPPY SCALE

AM	PM
1	1
2	2
3	3
4	4
5	5
6	6
7	7
8	8
9	9
10	10

NOTES / DOODLES

Get to know your breasts

DATE _____ **TIME** _____

Left	**Right**
Do you notice any changes?	**Do you notice any changes?**

Overall Breast Health

	Yes	No	If yes, what is different?
Bulging of skin	☐	☐	
Color	☐	☐	
Dimpling	☐	☐	
Puckering	☐	☐	
Shape	☐	☐	
Size	☐	☐	
Swelling	☐	☐	
Pain	☐	☐	1 2 3 4 5 6 7 8 9 10
Soreness	☐	☐	1 2 3 4 5 6 7 8 9 10

	Yes	No	If yes, what is different?
Bulging of skin	☐	☐	
Color	☐	☐	
Dimpling	☐	☐	
Puckering	☐	☐	
Shape	☐	☐	
Size	☐	☐	
Swelling	☐	☐	
Pain	☐	☐	1 2 3 4 5 6 7 8 9 10
Soreness	☐	☐	1 2 3 4 5 6 7 8 9 10

Nipple

Position	☐	☐
Ex: position change: Inward instead of pushing outward		
Redness	☐	☐
Ex: Position change: Inward instead of pushing outward		
Fluid	☐	☐
Ex: blood, milky, yellow fluid, or watery		

Position	☐	☐
Ex: position change: Inward instead of pushing outward		
Redness	☐	☐
Ex: Position change: Inward instead of pushing outward		
Fluid	☐	☐
Ex: blood, milky, yellow fluid, or watery		

Lump

Bulging of skin	☐	☐
Color	☐	☐
Dimpling	☐	☐

Bulging of skin	☐	☐
Color	☐	☐
Dimpling	☐	☐

Next steps: Notified Dr. ☐ Dr's Appointment ☐

Label lump, pain, and/or create your own label

USE L = LUMP **USE P = PAIN**

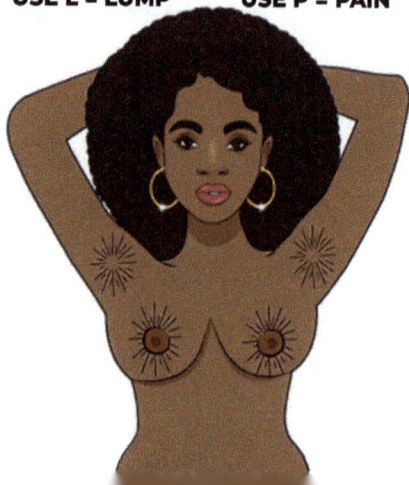

HAPPY SCALE

	AM	PM
	1	1
😐	2	2
	3	3
	4	4
🙂	5	5
	6	6
	7	7
😆	8	8
	9	9
	10	10

NOTES / DOODLES

Get to know your breasts

DATE _____ TIME _____

Left	Right
Do you notice any changes?	**Do you notice any changes?**

Overall Breast Health

	Yes	No	If yes, what is different?
Bulging of skin	☐	☐	
Color	☐	☐	
Dimpling	☐	☐	
Puckering	☐	☐	
Shape	☐	☐	
Size	☐	☐	
Swelling	☐	☐	
Pain	☐	☐	1 2 3 4 5 6 7 8 9 10
Soreness	☐	☐	1 2 3 4 5 6 7 8 9 10

	Yes	No	If yes, what is different?
Bulging of skin	☐	☐	
Color	☐	☐	
Dimpling	☐	☐	
Puckering	☐	☐	
Shape	☐	☐	
Size	☐	☐	
Swelling	☐	☐	
Pain	☐	☐	1 2 3 4 5 6 7 8 9 10
Soreness	☐	☐	1 2 3 4 5 6 7 8 9 10

Nipple

Position	☐	☐
Ex: position change: Inward instead of pushing outward		
Redness	☐	☐
Ex: Position change: Inward instead of pushing outward		
Fluid	☐	☐
Ex: blood, milky, yellow fluid, or watery		

Position	☐	☐
Ex: position change: Inward instead of pushing outward		
Redness	☐	☐
Ex: Position change: Inward instead of pushing outward		
Fluid	☐	☐
Ex: blood, milky, yellow fluid, or watery		

Lump

Bulging of skin	☐	☐
Color	☐	☐
Dimpling	☐	☐

Bulging of skin	☐	☐
Color	☐	☐
Dimpling	☐	☐

Next steps: Notified Dr. ☐   Dr's Appointment ☐

Label Lump, pain, and/or create your own label

USE L = LUMP   **USE P = PAIN**

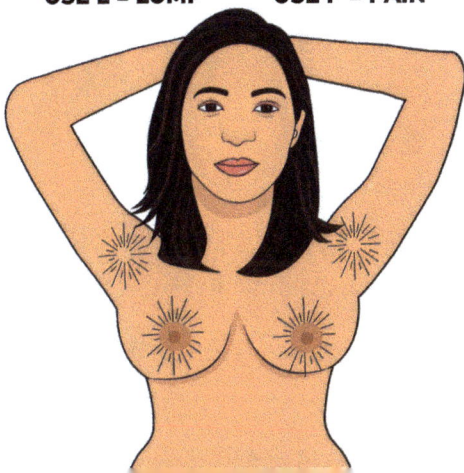

HAPPY SCALE

AM	PM
1	1
2	2
3	3
4	4
5	5
6	6
7	7
8	8
9	9
10	10

NOTES / DOODLES

55

Get to know your breasts

DATE _____   TIME _____

Left

Do you notice any changes?

Right

Do you notice any changes?

Overall Breast Health

	Yes	No	If yes, what is different?
Bulging of skin	☐	☐	
Color	☐	☐	
Dimpling	☐	☐	
Puckering	☐	☐	
Shape	☐	☐	
Size	☐	☐	
Swelling	☐	☐	
Pain	☐	☐	1 2 3 4 5 6 7 8 9 10
Soreness	☐	☐	1 2 3 4 5 6 7 8 9 10

	Yes	No	If yes, what is different?
Bulging of skin	☐	☐	
Color	☐	☐	
Dimpling	☐	☐	
Puckering	☐	☐	
Shape	☐	☐	
Size	☐	☐	
Swelling	☐	☐	
Pain	☐	☐	1 2 3 4 5 6 7 8 9 10
Soreness	☐	☐	1 2 3 4 5 6 7 8 9 10

Nipple

Position	☐	☐
Ex: position change: Inward instead of pushing outward		
Redness	☐	☐
Ex: Position change: Inward instead of pushing outward		
Fluid	☐	☐
Ex: blood, milky, yellow fluid, or watery		

Position	☐	☐
Ex: position change: Inward instead of pushing outward		
Redness	☐	☐
Ex: Position change: Inward instead of pushing outward		
Fluid	☐	☐
Ex: blood, milky, yellow fluid, or watery		

Lump

Bulging of skin	☐	☐
Color	☐	☐
Dimpling	☐	☐

Bulging of skin	☐	☐
Color	☐	☐
Dimpling	☐	☐

Next steps: Notified Dr. ☐   Dr's Appointment ☐

Label lump, pain, and/or create your own label

USE L = LUMP   **USE P = PAIN**

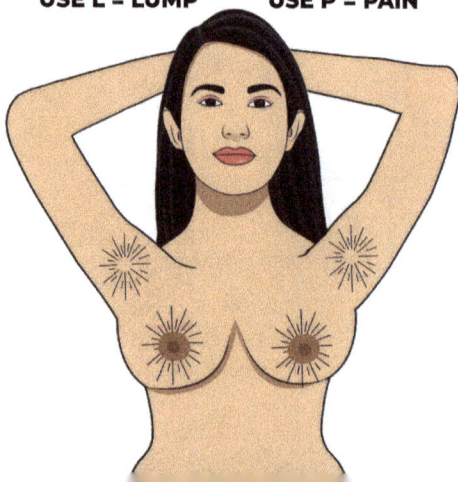

HAPPY SCALE

AM	PM
1	1
2	2
3	3
4	4
5	5
6	6
7	7
8	8
9	9
10	10

NOTES / DOODLES

Get to know your breasts

DATE _____ TIME _____

Left	Right
Do you notice any changes?	**Do you notice any changes?**

Overall Breast Health

	Yes	No	If yes, what is different?
Bulging of skin	☐	☐	
Color	☐	☐	
Dimpling	☐	☐	
Puckering	☐	☐	
Shape	☐	☐	
Size	☐	☐	
Swelling	☐	☐	
Pain	☐	☐	1 2 3 4 5 6 7 8 9 10
Soreness	☐	☐	1 2 3 4 5 6 7 8 9 10

	Yes	No	If yes, what is different?
Bulging of skin	☐	☐	
Color	☐	☐	
Dimpling	☐	☐	
Puckering	☐	☐	
Shape	☐	☐	
Size	☐	☐	
Swelling	☐	☐	
Pain	☐	☐	1 2 3 4 5 6 7 8 9 10
Soreness	☐	☐	1 2 3 4 5 6 7 8 9 10

Nipple

Left	Right
Position ☐ ☐	**Position** ☐ ☐
Ex: position change: Inward instead of pushing outward	*Ex: position change: Inward instead of pushing outward*
Redness ☐ ☐	**Redness** ☐ ☐
Ex: Position change: Inward instead of pushing outward	*Ex: Position change: Inward instead of pushing outward*
Fluid ☐ ☐	**Fluid** ☐ ☐
Ex: blood, milky, yellow fluid, or watery	*Ex: blood, milky, yellow fluid, or watery*

Lump

Left	Right
Bulging of skin ☐ ☐	Bulging of skin ☐ ☐
Color ☐ ☐	Color ☐ ☐
Dimpling ☐ ☐	Dimpling ☐ ☐

Next steps: Notified Dr. ☐   Dr's Appointment ☐

Label lump, pain, and/or create your own label

USE L = LUMP   **USE P = PAIN**

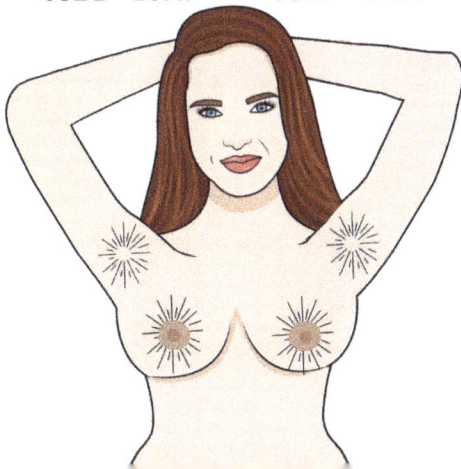

HAPPY SCALE

AM	PM
1	1
2	2
3	3
4	4
5	5
6	6
7	7
8	8
9	9
10	10

NOTES / DOODLES

Get to know your breasts

DATE _____   TIME _____

Left
Do you notice any changes?

Right
Do you notice any changes?

Overall Breast Health

	Yes	No	If yes, what is different?
Bulging of skin	☐	☐	
Color	☐	☐	
Dimpling	☐	☐	
Puckering	☐	☐	
Shape	☐	☐	
Size	☐	☐	
Swelling	☐	☐	
Pain	☐	☐	1 2 3 4 5 6 7 8 9 10
Soreness	☐	☐	1 2 3 4 5 6 7 8 9 10

	Yes	No	If yes, what is different?
Bulging of skin	☐	☐	
Color	☐	☐	
Dimpling	☐	☐	
Puckering	☐	☐	
Shape	☐	☐	
Size	☐	☐	
Swelling	☐	☐	
Pain	☐	☐	1 2 3 4 5 6 7 8 9 10
Soreness	☐	☐	1 2 3 4 5 6 7 8 9 10

Nipple

Position ☐ ☐
Ex: position change: Inward instead of pushing outward

Redness ☐ ☐
Ex: Position change: Inward instead of pushing outward

Fluid ☐ ☐
Ex: blood, milky, yellow fluid, or watery

Position ☐ ☐
Ex: position change: Inward instead of pushing outward

Redness ☐ ☐
Ex: Position change: Inward instead of pushing outward

Fluid ☐ ☐
Ex: blood, milky, yellow fluid, or watery

Lump

Bulging of skin	☐ ☐
Color	☐ ☐
Dimpling	☐ ☐

Bulging of skin	☐ ☐
Color	☐ ☐
Dimpling	☐ ☐

Next steps: Notified Dr. ☐   Dr's Appointment ☐

Label lump, pain, and/or create your own label

USE L = LUMP   **USE P = PAIN**

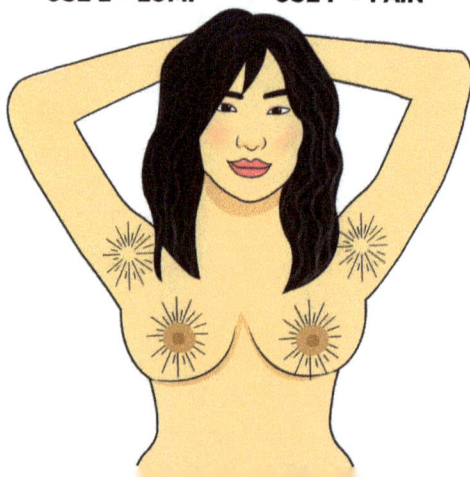

HAPPY SCALE

AM	PM
1	1
2	2
3	3
4	4
5	5
6	6
7	7
8	8
9	9
10	10

NOTES / DOODLES

Get to know your breasts

DATE _____ **TIME** _____

Left	Right
Do you notice any changes?	**Do you notice any changes?**

Overall Breast Health

Left

	Yes	No	If yes, what is different?
Bulging of skin	☐	☐	
Color	☐	☐	
Dimpling	☐	☐	
Puckering	☐	☐	
Shape	☐	☐	
Size	☐	☐	
Swelling	☐	☐	
Pain	☐	☐	1 2 3 4 5 6 7 8 9 10
Soreness	☐	☐	1 2 3 4 5 6 7 8 9 10

Right

	Yes	No	If yes, what is different?
Bulging of skin	☐	☐	
Color	☐	☐	
Dimpling	☐	☐	
Puckering	☐	☐	
Shape	☐	☐	
Size	☐	☐	
Swelling	☐	☐	
Pain	☐	☐	1 2 3 4 5 6 7 8 9 10
Soreness	☐	☐	1 2 3 4 5 6 7 8 9 10

Nipple

Left

Position	☐ ☐
Ex: position change: Inward instead of pushing outward	
Redness	☐ ☐
Ex: Position change: Inward instead of pushing outward	
Fluid	☐ ☐
Ex: blood, milky, yellow fluid, or watery	

Right

Position	☐ ☐
Ex: position change: Inward instead of pushing outward	
Redness	☐ ☐
Ex: Position change: Inward instead of pushing outward	
Fluid	☐ ☐
Ex: blood, milky, yellow fluid, or watery	

Lump

Left

Bulging of skin	☐ ☐
Color	☐ ☐
Dimpling	☐ ☐

Right

Bulging of skin	☐ ☐
Color	☐ ☐
Dimpling	☐ ☐

Next steps: Notified Dr. ☐   Dr's Appointment ☐

Label Lump, pain, and/or create your own label

USE L = LUMP   **USE P = PAIN**

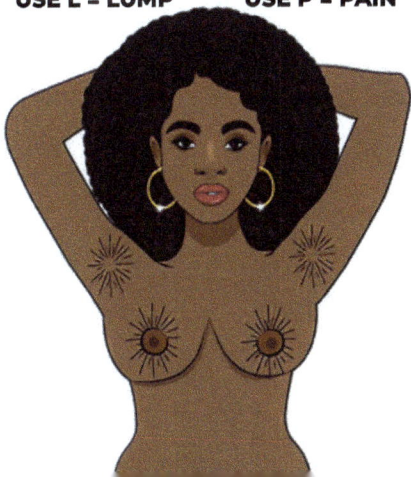

HAPPY SCALE

AM	PM
1	1
2	2
3	3
4	4
5	5
6	6
7	7
8	8
9	9
10	10

NOTES / DOODLES

Get to know your breasts

DATE _____   TIME _____

Left
Do you notice any changes?

Right
Do you notice any changes?

Overall Breast Health

	Yes	No	If yes, what is different?
Bulging of skin	☐	☐	
Color	☐	☐	
Dimpling	☐	☐	
Puckering	☐	☐	
Shape	☐	☐	
Size	☐	☐	
Swelling	☐	☐	
Pain	☐	☐	1 2 3 4 5 6 7 8 9 10
Soreness	☐	☐	1 2 3 4 5 6 7 8 9 10

	Yes	No	If yes, what is different?
Bulging of skin	☐	☐	
Color	☐	☐	
Dimpling	☐	☐	
Puckering	☐	☐	
Shape	☐	☐	
Size	☐	☐	
Swelling	☐	☐	
Pain	☐	☐	1 2 3 4 5 6 7 8 9 10
Soreness	☐	☐	1 2 3 4 5 6 7 8 9 10

Nipple

Position	☐	☐	

Ex: position change: Inward instead of pushing outward

Redness	☐	☐	

Ex: Position change: Inward instead of pushing outward

Fluid	☐	☐	

Ex: blood, milky, yellow fluid, or watery

Position	☐	☐	

Ex: position change: Inward instead of pushing outward

Redness	☐	☐	

Ex: Position change: Inward instead of pushing outward

Fluid	☐	☐	

Ex: blood, milky, yellow fluid, or watery

Lump

Bulging of skin	☐	☐
Color	☐	☐
Dimpling	☐	☐

Bulging of skin	☐	☐
Color	☐	☐
Dimpling	☐	☐

Next steps: Notified Dr. ☐   Dr's Appointment ☐

Label lump, pain, and/or create your own label
USE L = LUMP   **USE P = PAIN**

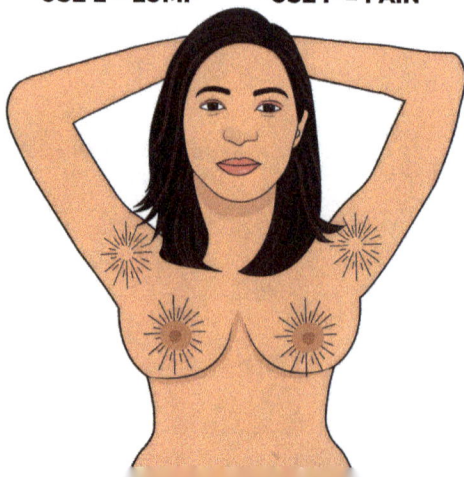

HAPPY SCALE

AM	PM
1	1
2	2
3	3
4	4
5	5
6	6
7	7
8	8
9	9
10	10

NOTES / DOODLES

Get to know your breasts

DATE ────────────────────────── TIME ──────────────────────────

Left
Do you notice any changes?

Right
Do you notice any changes?

Overall Breast Health

	Yes	No	If yes, what is different?
Bulging of skin	☐	☐	
Color	☐	☐	
Dimpling	☐	☐	
Puckering	☐	☐	
Shape	☐	☐	
Size	☐	☐	
Swelling	☐	☐	
Pain	☐	☐	1 2 3 4 5 6 7 8 9 10
Soreness	☐	☐	1 2 3 4 5 6 7 8 9 10

	Yes	No	If yes, what is different?
Bulging of skin	☐	☐	
Color	☐	☐	
Dimpling	☐	☐	
Puckering	☐	☐	
Shape	☐	☐	
Size	☐	☐	
Swelling	☐	☐	
Pain	☐	☐	1 2 3 4 5 6 7 8 9 10
Soreness	☐	☐	1 2 3 4 5 6 7 8 9 10

Nipple

Position ☐ ☐
Ex: position change: Inward instead of pushing outward

Redness ☐ ☐
Ex: Position change: Inward instead of pushing outward

Fluid ☐ ☐
Ex: blood, milky, yellow fluid, or watery

Position ☐ ☐
Ex: position change: Inward instead of pushing outward

Redness ☐ ☐
Ex: Position change: Inward instead of pushing outward

Fluid ☐ ☐
Ex: blood, milky, yellow fluid, or watery

Lump

Bulging of skin	☐ ☐
Color	☐ ☐
Dimpling	☐ ☐

Bulging of skin	☐ ☐
Color	☐ ☐
Dimpling	☐ ☐

Next steps: Notified Dr. ☐ Dr's Appointment ☐

Label Lump, pain, and/ or create your own label

USE L = LUMP **USE P = PAIN**

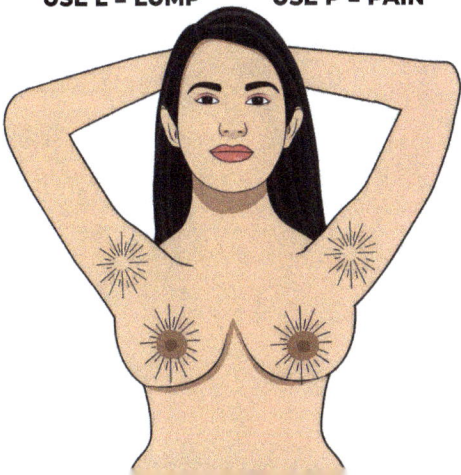

HAPPY SCALE

AM	PM
1	1
2	2
3	3
4	4
5	5
6	6
7	7
8	8
9	9
10	10

NOTES / DOODLES

Get to know your breasts

DATE _____ TIME _____

Left	Right
Do you notice any changes?	**Do you notice any changes?**

Overall Breast Health

	Yes	No	If yes, what is different?
Bulging of skin	☐	☐	
Color	☐	☐	
Dimpling	☐	☐	
Puckering	☐	☐	
Shape	☐	☐	
Size	☐	☐	
Swelling	☐	☐	
Pain	☐	☐	1 2 3 4 5 6 7 8 9 10
Soreness	☐	☐	1 2 3 4 5 6 7 8 9 10

	Yes	No	If yes, what is different?
Bulging of skin	☐	☐	
Color	☐	☐	
Dimpling	☐	☐	
Puckering	☐	☐	
Shape	☐	☐	
Size	☐	☐	
Swelling	☐	☐	
Pain	☐	☐	1 2 3 4 5 6 7 8 9 10
Soreness	☐	☐	1 2 3 4 5 6 7 8 9 10

Nipple

Position	☐ ☐	
Ex: position change: Inward instead of pushing outward		
Redness	☐ ☐	
Ex: Position change: Inward instead of pushing outward		
Fluid	☐ ☐	
Ex: blood, milky, yellow fluid, or watery		

Position	☐ ☐	
Ex: position change: Inward instead of pushing outward		
Redness	☐ ☐	
Ex: Position change: Inward instead of pushing outward		
Fluid	☐ ☐	
Ex: blood, milky, yellow fluid, or watery		

Lump

Bulging of skin	☐ ☐	
Color	☐ ☐	
Dimpling	☐ ☐	

Bulging of skin	☐ ☐	
Color	☐ ☐	
Dimpling	☐ ☐	

Next steps: Notified Dr. ☐   Dr's Appointment ☐

Label lump, pain, and/or create your own label
USE L = LUMP   **USE P = PAIN**

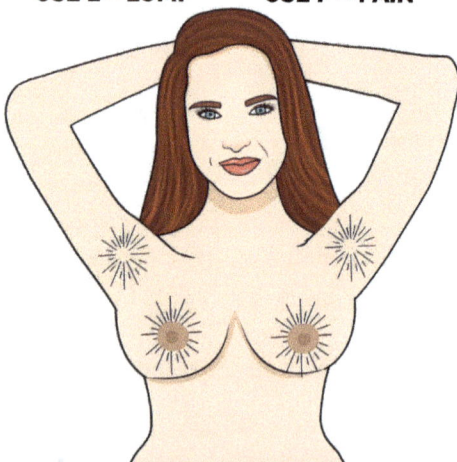

HAPPY SCALE

AM	PM
1	1
2	2
3	3
4	4
5	5
6	6
7	7
8	8
9	9
10	10

NOTES / DOODLES

Get to know your breasts

DATE _____ TIME _____

Left	Right
Do you notice any changes?	**Do you notice any changes?**

Overall Breast Health

	Yes	No	If yes, what is different?		Yes	No	If yes, what is different?
Bulging of skin	☐	☐		**Bulging of skin**	☐	☐	
Color	☐	☐		**Color**	☐	☐	
Dimpling	☐	☐		**Dimpling**	☐	☐	
Puckering	☐	☐		**Puckering**	☐	☐	
Shape	☐	☐		**Shape**	☐	☐	
Size	☐	☐		**Size**	☐	☐	
Swelling	☐	☐		**Swelling**	☐	☐	
Pain	☐	☐	1 2 3 4 5 6 7 8 9 10	**Pain**	☐	☐	1 2 3 4 5 6 7 8 9 10
Soreness	☐	☐	1 2 3 4 5 6 7 8 9 10	**Soreness**	☐	☐	1 2 3 4 5 6 7 8 9 10

Nipple

	Yes	No			Yes	No	
Position	☐	☐		**Position**	☐	☐	
Ex: position change: Inward instead of pushing outward				*Ex: position change: Inward instead of pushing outward*			
Redness	☐	☐		**Redness**	☐	☐	
Ex: Position change: Inward instead of pushing outward				*Ex: Position change: Inward instead of pushing outward*			
Fluid	☐	☐		**Fluid**	☐	☐	
Ex: blood, milky, yellow fluid, or watery				*Ex: blood, milky, yellow fluid, or watery*			

Lump

	Yes	No			Yes	No	
Bulging of skin	☐	☐		**Bulging of skin**	☐	☐	
Color	☐	☐		**Color**	☐	☐	
Dimpling	☐	☐		**Dimpling**	☐	☐	

Next steps: Notified Dr. ☐   Dr's Appointment ☐

Label Lump, pain, and/or create your own label

USE L = LUMP   USE P = PAIN

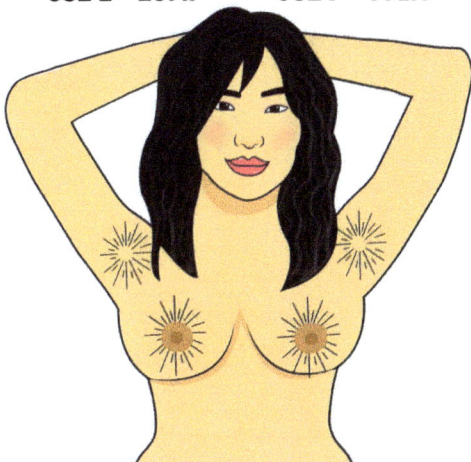

HAPPY SCALE

	AM	PM
	1	1
🙂	2	2
	3	3
	4	4
🙂	5	5
	6	6
	7	7
😆	8	8
	9	9
	10	10

NOTES / DOODLES

Get to know your breasts

DATE _____ TIME _____

Left	Right
Do you notice any changes?	**Do you notice any changes?**

Overall Breast Health

	Yes	No	If yes, what is different?
Bulging of skin	☐	☐	
Color	☐	☐	
Dimpling	☐	☐	
Puckering	☐	☐	
Shape	☐	☐	
Size	☐	☐	
Swelling	☐	☐	
Pain	☐	☐	1 2 3 4 5 6 7 8 9 10
Soreness	☐	☐	1 2 3 4 5 6 7 8 9 10

	Yes	No	If yes, what is different?
Bulging of skin	☐	☐	
Color	☐	☐	
Dimpling	☐	☐	
Puckering	☐	☐	
Shape	☐	☐	
Size	☐	☐	
Swelling	☐	☐	
Pain	☐	☐	1 2 3 4 5 6 7 8 9 10
Soreness	☐	☐	1 2 3 4 5 6 7 8 9 10

Nipple

Position	☐	☐
Ex: position change: Inward instead of pushing outward		
Redness	☐	☐
Ex: Position change: Inward instead of pushing outward		
Fluid	☐	☐
Ex: blood, milky, yellow fluid, or watery		

Position	☐	☐
Ex: position change: Inward instead of pushing outward		
Redness	☐	☐
Ex: Position change: Inward instead of pushing outward		
Fluid	☐	☐
Ex: blood, milky, yellow fluid, or watery		

Lump

Bulging of skin	☐	☐
Color	☐	☐
Dimpling	☐	☐

Bulging of skin	☐	☐
Color	☐	☐
Dimpling	☐	☐

Next steps: Notified Dr. ☐   Dr's Appointment ☐

Label Lump, pain, and/or create your own label
USE L = LUMP   **USE P = PAIN**

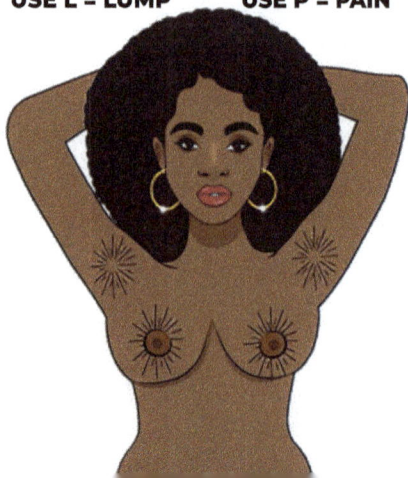

HAPPY SCALE

AM	PM
1	1
2	2
3	3
4	4
5	5
6	6
7	7
8	8
9	9
10	10

NOTES / DOODLES

Get to know your breasts

DATE _____ TIME _____

Left	Right
Do you notice any changes?	**Do you notice any changes?**

Overall Breast Health

	Yes	No	If yes, what is different?
Bulging of skin	☐	☐	
Color	☐	☐	
Dimpling	☐	☐	
Puckering	☐	☐	
Shape	☐	☐	
Size	☐	☐	
Swelling	☐	☐	
Pain	☐	☐	1 2 3 4 5 6 7 8 9 10
Soreness	☐	☐	1 2 3 4 5 6 7 8 9 10

	Yes	No	If yes, what is different?
Bulging of skin	☐	☐	
Color	☐	☐	
Dimpling	☐	☐	
Puckering	☐	☐	
Shape	☐	☐	
Size	☐	☐	
Swelling	☐	☐	
Pain	☐	☐	1 2 3 4 5 6 7 8 9 10
Soreness	☐	☐	1 2 3 4 5 6 7 8 9 10

Nipple

Position ☐ ☐
Ex: position change: Inward instead of pushing outward

Redness ☐ ☐
Ex: Position change: Inward instead of pushing outward

Fluid ☐ ☐
Ex: blood, milky, yellow fluid, or watery

Position ☐ ☐
Ex: position change: Inward instead of pushing outward

Redness ☐ ☐
Ex: Position change: Inward instead of pushing outward

Fluid ☐ ☐
Ex: blood, milky, yellow fluid, or watery

Lump

Bulging of skin	☐ ☐
Color	☐ ☐
Dimpling	☐ ☐

Bulging of skin	☐ ☐
Color	☐ ☐
Dimpling	☐ ☐

Next steps: Notified Dr. ☐   Dr's Appointment ☐

Label lump, pain, and/or create your own label

USE L = LUMP   **USE P = PAIN**

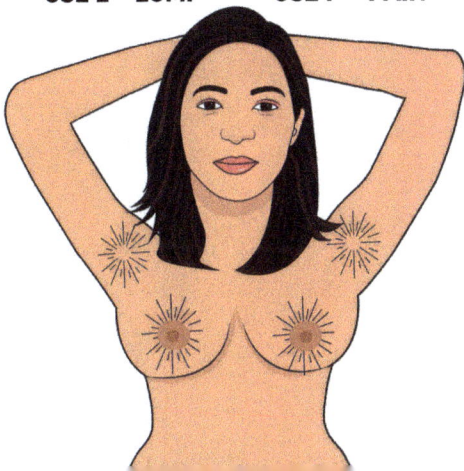

HAPPY SCALE

AM	PM
1	1
2	2
3	3
4	4
5	5
6	6
7	7
8	8
9	9
10	10

NOTES / DOODLES

Get to know your breasts

DATE _____ **TIME** _____

Left
Do you notice any changes?

Right
Do you notice any changes?

Overall Breast Health

Left

	Yes	No	If yes, what is different?
Bulging of skin	☐	☐	
Color	☐	☐	
Dimpling	☐	☐	
Puckering	☐	☐	
Shape	☐	☐	
Size	☐	☐	
Swelling	☐	☐	
Pain	☐	☐	1 2 3 4 5 6 7 8 9 10
Soreness	☐	☐	1 2 3 4 5 6 7 8 9 10

Right

	Yes	No	If yes, what is different?
Bulging of skin	☐	☐	
Color	☐	☐	
Dimpling	☐	☐	
Puckering	☐	☐	
Shape	☐	☐	
Size	☐	☐	
Swelling	☐	☐	
Pain	☐	☐	1 2 3 4 5 6 7 8 9 10
Soreness	☐	☐	1 2 3 4 5 6 7 8 9 10

Nipple

Left

Position	☐	☐
Ex: position change: Inward instead of pushing outward		
Redness	☐	☐
Ex: Position change: Inward instead of pushing outward		
Fluid	☐	☐
Ex: blood, milky, yellow fluid, or watery		

Right

Position	☐	☐
Ex: position change: Inward instead of pushing outward		
Redness	☐	☐
Ex: Position change: Inward instead of pushing outward		
Fluid	☐	☐
Ex: blood, milky, yellow fluid, or watery		

Lump

Left

Bulging of skin	☐	☐
Color	☐	☐
Dimpling	☐	☐

Right

Bulging of skin	☐	☐
Color	☐	☐
Dimpling	☐	☐

Next steps: Notified Dr. ☐   Dr's Appointment ☐

Label lump, pain, and/or create your own label

USE L = LUMP   **USE P = PAIN**

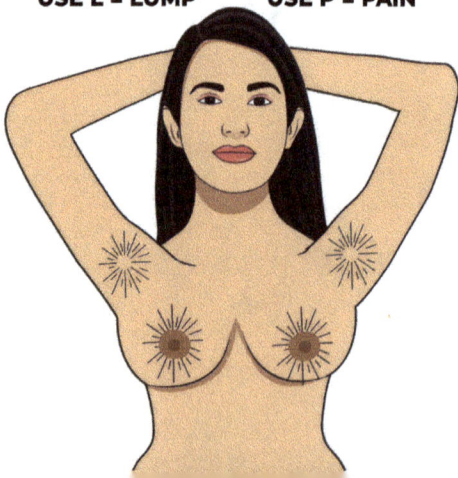

HAPPY SCALE

AM	PM
1	1
2	2
3	3
4	4
5	5
6	6
7	7
8	8
9	9
10	10

NOTES / DOODLES

Get to know your breasts

DATE _____ **TIME** _____

Left	Right
Do you notice any changes?	**Do you notice any changes?**

Overall Breast Health

	Yes	No	If yes, what is different?			Yes	No	If yes, what is different?
Bulging of skin	☐	☐			**Bulging of skin**	☐	☐	
Color	☐	☐			**Color**	☐	☐	
Dimpling	☐	☐			**Dimpling**	☐	☐	
Puckering	☐	☐			**Puckering**	☐	☐	
Shape	☐	☐			**Shape**	☐	☐	
Size	☐	☐			**Size**	☐	☐	
Swelling	☐	☐			**Swelling**	☐	☐	
Pain	☐	☐	1 2 3 4 5 6 7 8 9 10		**Pain**	☐	☐	1 2 3 4 5 6 7 8 9 10
Soreness	☐	☐	1 2 3 4 5 6 7 8 9 10		**Soreness**	☐	☐	1 2 3 4 5 6 7 8 9 10

Nipple

Position ☐ ☐				**Position** ☐ ☐			
Ex: position change: Inward instead of pushing outward				*Ex: position change: Inward instead of pushing outward*			
Redness ☐ ☐				**Redness** ☐ ☐			
Ex: Position change: Inward instead of pushing outward				*Ex: Position change: Inward instead of pushing outward*			
Fluid ☐ ☐				**Fluid** ☐ ☐			
Ex: blood, milky, yellow fluid, or watery				*Ex: blood, milky, yellow fluid, or watery*			

Lump

Bulging of skin ☐ ☐		**Bulging of skin** ☐ ☐	
Color ☐ ☐		**Color** ☐ ☐	
Dimpling ☐ ☐		**Dimpling** ☐ ☐	

Next steps: Notified Dr. ☐   Dr's Appointment ☐

Label Lump, pain, and/or create your own label

USE L = LUMP   **USE P = PAIN**

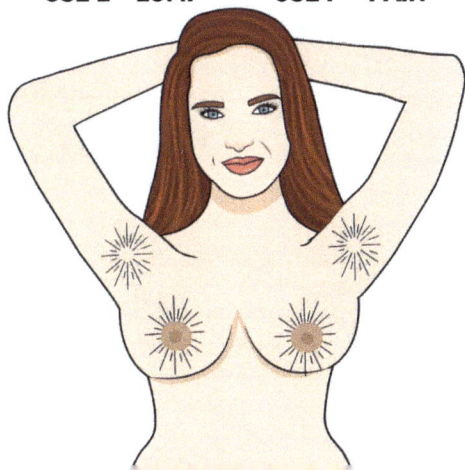

HAPPY SCALE

AM	PM
1	1
2	2
3	3
4	4
5	5
6	6
7	7
8	8
9	9
10	10

NOTES / DOODLES

Get to know your breasts

DATE _____ TIME _____

Left	Right
Do you notice any changes?	**Do you notice any changes?**

Overall Breast Health

	Yes	No	If yes, what is different?
Bulging of skin	☐	☐	
Color	☐	☐	
Dimpling	☐	☐	
Puckering	☐	☐	
Shape	☐	☐	
Size	☐	☐	
Swelling	☐	☐	
Pain	☐	☐	1 2 3 4 5 6 7 8 9 10
Soreness	☐	☐	1 2 3 4 5 6 7 8 9 10

	Yes	No	If yes, what is different?
Bulging of skin	☐	☐	
Color	☐	☐	
Dimpling	☐	☐	
Puckering	☐	☐	
Shape	☐	☐	
Size	☐	☐	
Swelling	☐	☐	
Pain	☐	☐	1 2 3 4 5 6 7 8 9 10
Soreness	☐	☐	1 2 3 4 5 6 7 8 9 10

Nipple

Position ☐ ☐
Ex: position change: Inward instead of pushing outward

Redness ☐ ☐
Ex: Position change: Inward instead of pushing outward

Fluid ☐ ☐
Ex: blood, milky, yellow fluid, or watery

Position ☐ ☐
Ex: position change: Inward instead of pushing outward

Redness ☐ ☐
Ex: Position change: Inward instead of pushing outward

Fluid ☐ ☐
Ex: blood, milky, yellow fluid, or watery

Lump

Bulging of skin	☐ ☐
Color	☐ ☐
Dimpling	☐ ☐

Bulging of skin	☐ ☐
Color	☐ ☐
Dimpling	☐ ☐

Next steps: Notified Dr. ☐   Dr's Appointment ☐

Label lump, pain, and/or create your own label
USE L = LUMP   **USE P = PAIN**

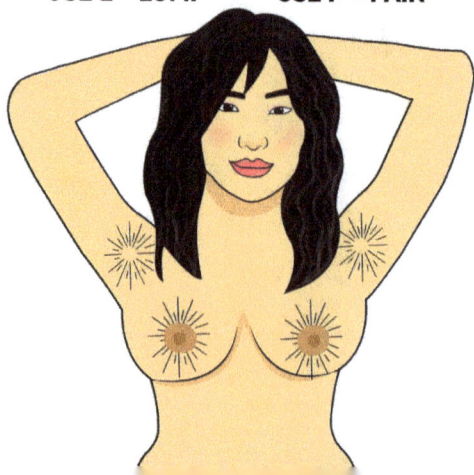

HAPPY SCALE

AM	PM
1	1
2	2
3	3
4	4
5	5
6	6
7	7
8	8
9	9
10	10

NOTES / DOODLES

Get to know your breasts

DATE _____ TIME _____

Left	Right
Do you notice any changes?	**Do you notice any changes?**

Overall Breast Health

	Yes	No	If yes, what is different?
Bulging of skin	☐	☐	
Color	☐	☐	
Dimpling	☐	☐	
Puckering	☐	☐	
Shape	☐	☐	
Size	☐	☐	
Swelling	☐	☐	
Pain	☐	☐	1 2 3 4 5 6 7 8 9 10
Soreness	☐	☐	1 2 3 4 5 6 7 8 9 10

	Yes	No	If yes, what is different?
Bulging of skin	☐	☐	
Color	☐	☐	
Dimpling	☐	☐	
Puckering	☐	☐	
Shape	☐	☐	
Size	☐	☐	
Swelling	☐	☐	
Pain	☐	☐	1 2 3 4 5 6 7 8 9 10
Soreness	☐	☐	1 2 3 4 5 6 7 8 9 10

Nipple

Position ☐ ☐
Ex: position change: Inward instead of pushing outward

Redness ☐ ☐
Ex: Position change: Inward instead of pushing outward

Fluid ☐ ☐
Ex: blood, milky, yellow fluid, or watery

Position ☐ ☐
Ex: position change: Inward instead of pushing outward

Redness ☐ ☐
Ex: Position change: Inward instead of pushing outward

Fluid ☐ ☐
Ex: blood, milky, yellow fluid, or watery

Lump

Bulging of skin ☐ ☐
Color ☐ ☐
Dimpling ☐ ☐

Bulging of skin ☐ ☐
Color ☐ ☐
Dimpling ☐ ☐

Next steps: Notified Dr. ☐   Dr's Appointment ☐

Label Lump, pain, and/or create your own label

USE L = LUMP   **USE P = PAIN**

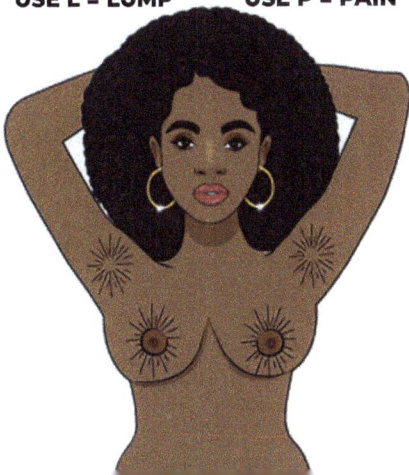

HAPPY SCALE

AM	PM
1	1
2	2
3	3
4	4
5	5
6	6
7	7
8	8
9	9
10	10

NOTES / DOODLES

Get to know your breasts

DATE _____   TIME _____

Left	Right
Do you notice any changes?	**Do you notice any changes?**

Overall Breast Health

	Yes	No	If yes, what is different?
Bulging of skin	☐	☐	
Color	☐	☐	
Dimpling	☐	☐	
Puckering	☐	☐	
Shape	☐	☐	
Size	☐	☐	
Swelling	☐	☐	
Pain	☐	☐	1 2 3 4 5 6 7 8 9 10
Soreness	☐	☐	1 2 3 4 5 6 7 8 9 10

	Yes	No	If yes, what is different?
Bulging of skin	☐	☐	
Color	☐	☐	
Dimpling	☐	☐	
Puckering	☐	☐	
Shape	☐	☐	
Size	☐	☐	
Swelling	☐	☐	
Pain	☐	☐	1 2 3 4 5 6 7 8 9 10
Soreness	☐	☐	1 2 3 4 5 6 7 8 9 10

Nipple

Left			
Position	☐	☐	
Ex: position change: Inward instead of pushing outward			
Redness	☐	☐	
Ex: Position change: Inward instead of pushing outward			
Fluid	☐	☐	
Ex: blood, milky, yellow fluid, or watery			

Right			
Position	☐	☐	
Ex: position change: Inward instead of pushing outward			
Redness	☐	☐	
Ex: Position change: Inward instead of pushing outward			
Fluid	☐	☐	
Ex: blood, milky, yellow fluid, or watery			

Lump

Bulging of skin	☐	☐	
Color	☐	☐	
Dimpling	☐	☐	

Bulging of skin	☐	☐	
Color	☐	☐	
Dimpling	☐	☐	

Next steps: Notified Dr. ☐   Dr's Appointment ☐

Label lump, pain, and/or create your own label
USE L = LUMP   USE P = PAIN

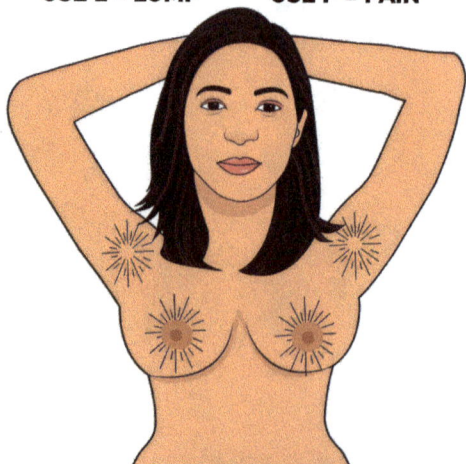

HAPPY SCALE

AM	PM
1	1
2	2
3	3
4	4
5	5
6	6
7	7
8	8
9	9
10	10

NOTES / DOODLES

Get to know your breasts

DATE _____ TIME _____

Left	Right
Do you notice any changes?	**Do you notice any changes?**

Overall Breast Health

	Yes	No	If yes, what is different?
Bulging of skin	☐	☐	
Color	☐	☐	
Dimpling	☐	☐	
Puckering	☐	☐	
Shape	☐	☐	
Size	☐	☐	
Swelling	☐	☐	
Pain	☐	☐	1 2 3 4 5 6 7 8 9 10
Soreness	☐	☐	1 2 3 4 5 6 7 8 9 10

	Yes	No	If yes, what is different?
Bulging of skin	☐	☐	
Color	☐	☐	
Dimpling	☐	☐	
Puckering	☐	☐	
Shape	☐	☐	
Size	☐	☐	
Swelling	☐	☐	
Pain	☐	☐	1 2 3 4 5 6 7 8 9 10
Soreness	☐	☐	1 2 3 4 5 6 7 8 9 10

Nipple

Position	☐	☐

Ex: position change: Inward instead of pushing outward

Redness	☐	☐

Ex: Position change: Inward instead of pushing outward

Fluid	☐	☐

Ex: blood, milky, yellow fluid, or watery

Position	☐	☐

Ex: position change: Inward instead of pushing outward

Redness	☐	☐

Ex: Position change: Inward instead of pushing outward

Fluid	☐	☐

Ex: blood, milky, yellow fluid, or watery

Lump

Bulging of skin	☐ ☐
Color	☐ ☐
Dimpling	☐ ☐

Bulging of skin	☐ ☐
Color	☐ ☐
Dimpling	☐ ☐

Next steps: Notified Dr. ☐   Dr's Appointment ☐

Label lump, pain, and/or create your own label

USE L = LUMP   **USE P = PAIN**

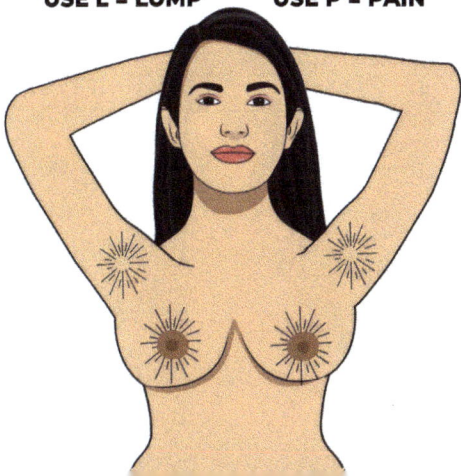

HAPPY SCALE

AM	PM
1	1
2	2
3	3
4	4
5	5
6	6
7	7
8	8
9	9
10	10

NOTES / DOODLES

71

Get to know your breasts

DATE _____   TIME _____

Left	Right
Do you notice any changes?	**Do you notice any changes?**

Overall Breast Health

Left	Yes	No	If yes, what is different?	Right	Yes	No	If yes, what is different?
Bulging of skin	☐	☐		Bulging of skin	☐	☐	
Color	☐	☐		Color	☐	☐	
Dimpling	☐	☐		Dimpling	☐	☐	
Puckering	☐	☐		Puckering	☐	☐	
Shape	☐	☐		Shape	☐	☐	
Size	☐	☐		Size	☐	☐	
Swelling	☐	☐		Swelling	☐	☐	
Pain	☐	☐	1 2 3 4 5 6 7 8 9 10	Pain	☐	☐	1 2 3 4 5 6 7 8 9 10
Soreness	☐	☐	1 2 3 4 5 6 7 8 9 10	Soreness	☐	☐	1 2 3 4 5 6 7 8 9 10

Nipple

Left			Right		
Position	☐	☐	Position	☐	☐
Ex: position change: Inward instead of pushing outward			*Ex: position change: Inward instead of pushing outward*		
Redness	☐	☐	Redness	☐	☐
Ex: Position change: Inward instead of pushing outward			*Ex: Position change: Inward instead of pushing outward*		
Fluid	☐	☐	Fluid	☐	☐
Ex: blood, milky, yellow fluid, or watery			*Ex: blood, milky, yellow fluid, or watery*		

Lump

Left			Right		
Bulging of skin	☐	☐	Bulging of skin	☐	☐
Color	☐	☐	Color	☐	☐
Dimpling	☐	☐	Dimpling	☐	☐

Next steps: Notified Dr. ☐   Dr's Appointment ☐

Label lump, pain, and/or create your own label

USE L = LUMP   **USE P = PAIN**

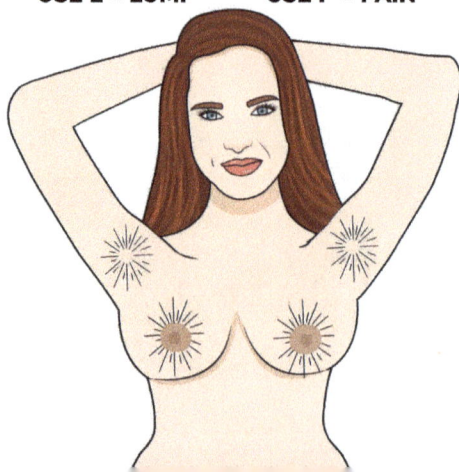

HAPPY SCALE

AM	PM
1	1
2	2
3	3
4	4
5	5
6	6
7	7
8	8
9	9
10	10

NOTES / DOODLES

Get to know your breasts

DATE _____   TIME _____

Left	Right
Do you notice any changes?	**Do you notice any changes?**

Overall Breast Health

	Yes	No	If yes, what is different?			Yes	No	If yes, what is different?
Bulging of skin	☐	☐			**Bulging of skin**	☐	☐	
Color	☐	☐			Color	☐	☐	
Dimpling	☐	☐			**Dimpling**	☐	☐	
Puckering	☐	☐			**Puckering**	☐	☐	
Shape	☐	☐			**Shape**	☐	☐	
Size	☐	☐			Size	☐	☐	
Swelling	☐	☐			**Swelling**	☐	☐	
Pain	☐	☐	1 2 3 4 5 6 7 8 9 10		Pain	☐	☐	1 2 3 4 5 6 7 8 9 10
Soreness	☐	☐	1 2 3 4 5 6 7 8 9 10		**Soreness**	☐	☐	1 2 3 4 5 6 7 8 9 10

Nipple

Position	☐	☐		**Position**	☐	☐	
Ex: position change: Inward instead of pushing outward				*Ex: position change: Inward instead of pushing outward*			
Redness	☐	☐		**Redness**	☐	☐	
Ex: Position change: Inward instead of pushing outward				*Ex: Position change: Inward instead of pushing outward*			
Fluid	☐	☐		**Fluid**	☐	☐	
Ex: blood, milky, yellow fluid, or watery				*Ex: blood, milky, yellow fluid, or watery*			

Lump

Bulging of skin	☐	☐		**Bulging of skin**	☐	☐
Color	☐	☐		**Color**	☐	☐
Dimpling	☐	☐		**Dimpling**	☐	☐

Next steps: Notified Dr. ☐   Dr's Appointment ☐

Label lump, pain, and/or create your own label

USE L = LUMP   **USE P = PAIN**

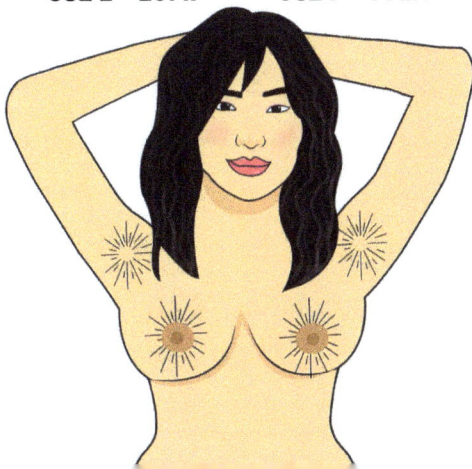

HAPPY SCALE

AM	PM
1	1
2	2
3	3
4	4
5	5
6	6
7	7
8	8
9	9
10	10

NOTES / DOODLES

Get to know your breasts

DATE _____ **TIME** _____

Left

Do you notice any changes?

Right

Do you notice any changes?

Overall Breast Health

	Yes	No	If yes, what is different?
Bulging of skin	☐	☐	
Color	☐	☐	
Dimpling	☐	☐	
Puckering	☐	☐	
Shape	☐	☐	
Size	☐	☐	
Swelling	☐	☐	
Pain	☐	☐	1 2 3 4 5 6 7 8 9 10
Soreness	☐	☐	1 2 3 4 5 6 7 8 9 10

	Yes	No	If yes, what is different?
Bulging of skin	☐	☐	
Color	☐	☐	
Dimpling	☐	☐	
Puckering	☐	☐	
Shape	☐	☐	
Size	☐	☐	
Swelling	☐	☐	
Pain	☐	☐	1 2 3 4 5 6 7 8 9 10
Soreness	☐	☐	1 2 3 4 5 6 7 8 9 10

Nipple

Position	☐ ☐	
Ex: position change: Inward instead of pushing outward		
Redness	☐ ☐	
Ex: Position change: Inward instead of pushing outward		
Fluid	☐ ☐	
Ex: blood, milky, yellow fluid, or watery		

Position	☐ ☐	
Ex: position change: Inward instead of pushing outward		
Redness	☐ ☐	
Ex: Position change: Inward instead of pushing outward		
Fluid	☐ ☐	
Ex: blood, milky, yellow fluid, or watery		

Lump

Bulging of skin	☐ ☐	
Color	☐ ☐	
Dimpling	☐ ☐	

Bulging of skin	☐ ☐	
Color	☐ ☐	
Dimpling	☐ ☐	

Next steps: Notified Dr. ☐   Dr's Appointment ☐

Label lump, pain, and/ or create your own label
USE L = LUMP   USE P = PAIN

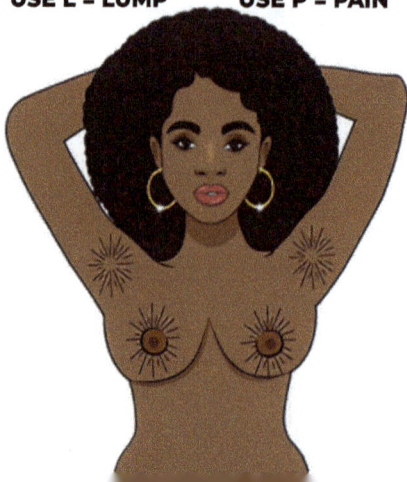

HAPPY SCALE

AM	PM
1	1
2	2
3	3
4	4
5	5
6	6
7	7
8	8
9	9
10	10

NOTES / DOODLES

Get to know your breasts

DATE _____ **TIME** _____

Left	Right
Do you notice any changes?	**Do you notice any changes?**

Overall Breast Health

	Yes	No	If yes, what is different?		Yes	No	If yes, what is different?
Bulging of skin	☐	☐		**Bulging of skin**	☐	☐	
Color	☐	☐		**Color**	☐	☐	
Dimpling	☐	☐		**Dimpling**	☐	☐	
Puckering	☐	☐		**Puckering**	☐	☐	
Shape	☐	☐		**Shape**	☐	☐	
Size	☐	☐		**Size**	☐	☐	
Swelling	☐	☐		**Swelling**	☐	☐	
Pain	☐	☐	1 2 3 4 5 6 7 8 9 10	**Pain**	☐	☐	1 2 3 4 5 6 7 8 9 10
Soreness	☐	☐	1 2 3 4 5 6 7 8 9 10	**Soreness**	☐	☐	1 2 3 4 5 6 7 8 9 10

Nipple

	Yes	No			Yes	No
Position	☐	☐		**Position**	☐	☐
Ex: position change: Inward instead of pushing outward				*Ex: position change: Inward instead of pushing outward*		
Redness	☐	☐		**Redness**	☐	☐
Ex: Position change: Inward instead of pushing outward				*Ex: Position change: Inward instead of pushing outward*		
Fluid	☐	☐		**Fluid**	☐	☐
Ex: blood, milky, yellow fluid, or watery				*Ex: blood, milky, yellow fluid, or watery*		

Lump

	Yes	No			Yes	No
Bulging of skin	☐	☐		**Bulging of skin**	☐	☐
Color	☐	☐		**Color**	☐	☐
Dimpling	☐	☐		**Dimpling**	☐	☐

Next steps: Notified Dr. ☐   Dr's Appointment ☐

Label Lump, pain, and/or create your own label

USE L = LUMP   **USE P = PAIN**

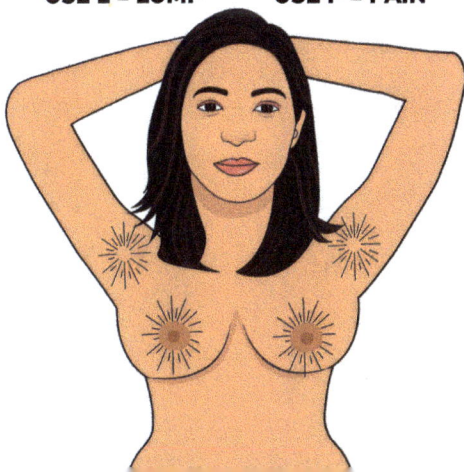

HAPPY SCALE

AM	PM
1	1
2	2
3	3
4	4
5	5
6	6
7	7
8	8
9	9
10	10

NOTES / DOODLES

Get to know your breasts

DATE _____ TIME _____

Left	Right
Do you notice any changes?	**Do you notice any changes?**

Overall Breast Health

	Yes	No	If yes, what is different?
Bulging of skin	☐	☐	
Color	☐	☐	
Dimpling	☐	☐	
Puckering	☐	☐	
Shape	☐	☐	
Size	☐	☐	
Swelling	☐	☐	
Pain	☐	☐	1 2 3 4 5 6 7 8 9 10
Soreness	☐	☐	1 2 3 4 5 6 7 8 9 10

	Yes	No	If yes, what is different?
Bulging of skin	☐	☐	
Color	☐	☐	
Dimpling	☐	☐	
Puckering	☐	☐	
Shape	☐	☐	
Size	☐	☐	
Swelling	☐	☐	
Pain	☐	☐	1 2 3 4 5 6 7 8 9 10
Soreness	☐	☐	1 2 3 4 5 6 7 8 9 10

Nipple

Position	☐	☐	

Ex: position change: Inward instead of pushing outward

Redness	☐	☐	

Ex: Position change: Inward instead of pushing outward

Fluid	☐	☐	

Ex: blood, milky, yellow fluid, or watery

Position	☐	☐	

Ex: position change: Inward instead of pushing outward

Redness	☐	☐	

Ex: Position change: Inward instead of pushing outward

Fluid	☐	☐	

Ex: blood, milky, yellow fluid, or watery

Lump

Bulging of skin	☐	☐
Color	☐	☐
Dimpling	☐	☐

Bulging of skin	☐	☐
Color	☐	☐
Dimpling	☐	☐

Next steps: Notified Dr. ☐   Dr's Appointment ☐

Label lump, pain, and/or create your own label

USE L = LUMP   **USE P = PAIN**

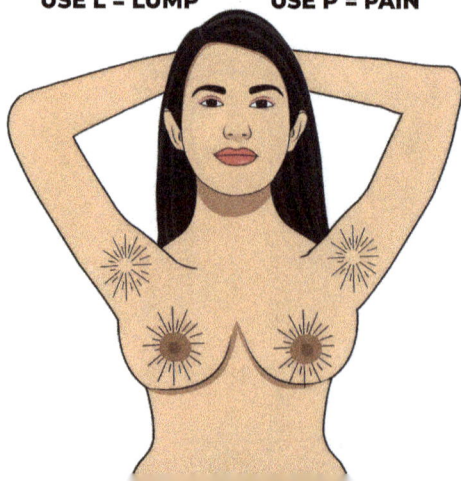

HAPPY SCALE

AM	PM
1	1
2	2
3	3
4	4
5	5
6	6
7	7
8	8
9	9
10	10

NOTES / DOODLES

Get to know your breasts

DATE _____   TIME _____

Left	Right
Do you notice any changes?	**Do you notice any changes?**

Overall Breast Health

	Yes	No	If yes, what is different?
Bulging of skin	☐	☐	
Color	☐	☐	
Dimpling	☐	☐	
Puckering	☐	☐	
Shape	☐	☐	
Size	☐	☐	
Swelling	☐	☐	
Pain	☐	☐	1 2 3 4 5 6 7 8 9 10
Soreness	☐	☐	1 2 3 4 5 6 7 8 9 10

	Yes	No	If yes, what is different?
Bulging of skin	☐	☐	
Color	☐	☐	
Dimpling	☐	☐	
Puckering	☐	☐	
Shape	☐	☐	
Size	☐	☐	
Swelling	☐	☐	
Pain	☐	☐	1 2 3 4 5 6 7 8 9 10
Soreness	☐	☐	1 2 3 4 5 6 7 8 9 10

Nipple

Position ☐ ☐

Ex: position change: Inward instead of pushing outward

Redness ☐ ☐

Ex: Position change: Inward instead of pushing outward

Fluid ☐ ☐

Ex: blood, milky, yellow fluid, or watery

Position ☐ ☐

Ex: position change: Inward instead of pushing outward

Redness ☐ ☐

Ex: Position change: Inward instead of pushing outward

Fluid ☐ ☐

Ex: blood, milky, yellow fluid, or watery

Lump

Bulging of skin	☐	☐
Color	☐	☐
Dimpling	☐	☐

Bulging of skin	☐	☐
Color	☐	☐
Dimpling	☐	☐

Next steps: Notified Dr. ☐   Dr's Appointment ☐

Label Lump, pain, and/or create your own label

USE L = LUMP   **USE P = PAIN**

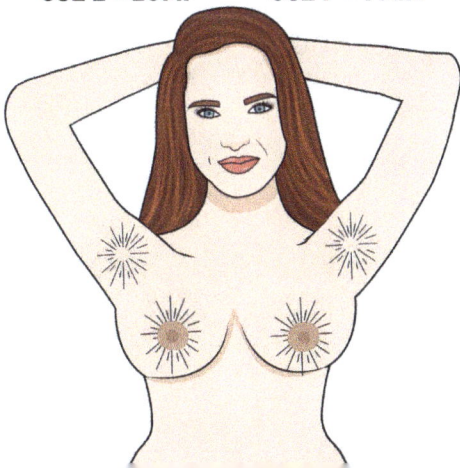

HAPPY SCALE

AM	PM
1	1
2	2
3	3
4	4
5	5
6	6
7	7
8	8
9	9
10	10

NOTES / DOODLES

Get to know your breasts

DATE ———————————————— TIME ————————————————

| **Left** | **Right** |

Do you notice any changes?   **Do you notice any changes?**

Overall Breast Health

	Yes	No	If yes, what is different?
Bulging of skin	☐	☐	
Color	☐	☐	
Dimpling	☐	☐	
Puckering	☐	☐	
Shape	☐	☐	
Size	☐	☐	
Swelling	☐	☐	
Pain	☐	☐	1 2 3 4 5 6 7 8 9 10
Soreness	☐	☐	1 2 3 4 5 6 7 8 9 10

	Yes	No	If yes, what is different?
Bulging of skin	☐	☐	
Color	☐	☐	
Dimpling	☐	☐	
Puckering	☐	☐	
Shape	☐	☐	
Size	☐	☐	
Swelling	☐	☐	
Pain	☐	☐	1 2 3 4 5 6 7 8 9 10
Soreness	☐	☐	1 2 3 4 5 6 7 8 9 10

Nipple

Position	☐ ☐
Ex: position change: Inward instead of pushing outward	
Redness	☐ ☐
Ex: Position change: Inward instead of pushing outward	
Fluid	☐ ☐
Ex: blood, milky, yellow fluid, or watery	

Position	☐ ☐
Ex: position change: Inward instead of pushing outward	
Redness	☐ ☐
Ex: Position change: Inward instead of pushing outward	
Fluid	☐ ☐
Ex: blood, milky, yellow fluid, or watery	

Lump

Bulging of skin	☐ ☐
Color	☐ ☐
Dimpling	☐ ☐

Bulging of skin	☐ ☐
Color	☐ ☐
Dimpling	☐ ☐

Next steps: Notified Dr. ☐   Dr's Appointment ☐

Label lump, pain, and/or create your own label

USE L = LUMP   **USE P = PAIN**

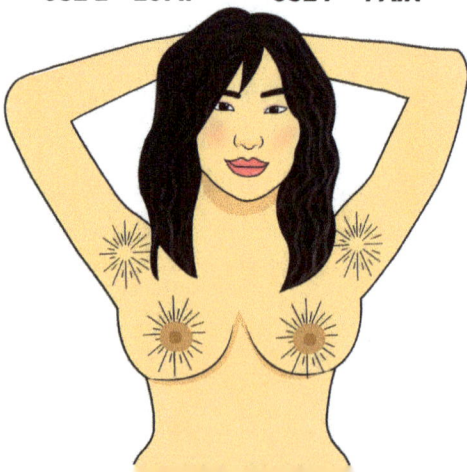

HAPPY SCALE

AM	PM
1	1
2	2
3	3
4	4
5	5
6	6
7	7
8	8
9	9
10	10

NOTES / DOODLES

Get to know your breasts

DATE _____   **TIME** _____

Left	Right
Do you notice any changes?	**Do you notice any changes?**

Overall Breast Health

Left

	Yes	No	If yes, what is different?
Bulging of skin	☐	☐	
Color	☐	☐	
Dimpling	☐	☐	
Puckering	☐	☐	
Shape	☐	☐	
Size	☐	☐	
Swelling	☐	☐	
Pain	☐	☐	1 2 3 4 5 6 7 8 9 10
Soreness	☐	☐	1 2 3 4 5 6 7 8 9 10

Right

	Yes	No	If yes, what is different?
Bulging of skin	☐	☐	
Color	☐	☐	
Dimpling	☐	☐	
Puckering	☐	☐	
Shape	☐	☐	
Size	☐	☐	
Swelling	☐	☐	
Pain	☐	☐	1 2 3 4 5 6 7 8 9 10
Soreness	☐	☐	1 2 3 4 5 6 7 8 9 10

Nipple

Left

Position	☐	☐

Ex: position change: Inward instead of pushing outward

Redness	☐	☐

Ex: Position change: Inward instead of pushing outward

Fluid	☐	☐

Ex: blood, milky, yellow fluid, or watery

Right

Position	☐	☐

Ex: position change: Inward instead of pushing outward

Redness	☐	☐

Ex: Position change: Inward instead of pushing outward

Fluid	☐	☐

Ex: blood, milky, yellow fluid, or watery

Lump

Left

Bulging of skin	☐	☐
Color	☐	☐
Dimpling	☐	☐

Right

Bulging of skin	☐	☐
Color	☐	☐
Dimpling	☐	☐

Next steps: Notified Dr. ☐   Dr's Appointment ☐

Label lump, pain, and/or create your own label

USE L = LUMP   **USE P = PAIN**

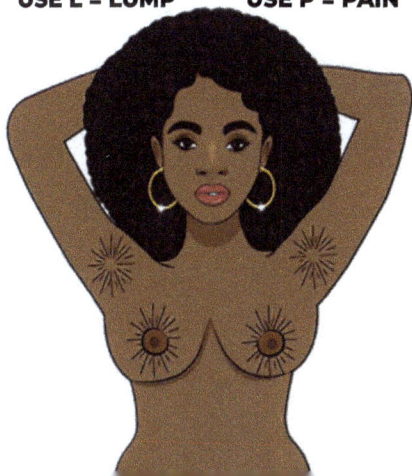

HAPPY SCALE

AM	PM
1	1
2	2
3	3
4	4
5	5
6	6
7	7
8	8
9	9
10	10

NOTES / DOODLES

Get to know your breasts

DATE _____   TIME _____

	Left		Right
	Do you notice any changes?		**Do you notice any changes?**

Overall Breast Health

	Yes	No	If yes, what is different?
Bulging of skin	☐	☐	
Color	☐	☐	
Dimpling	☐	☐	
Puckering	☐	☐	
Shape	☐	☐	
Size	☐	☐	
Swelling	☐	☐	
Pain	☐	☐	1 2 3 4 5 6 7 8 9 10
Soreness	☐	☐	1 2 3 4 5 6 7 8 9 10

	Yes	No	If yes, what is different?
Bulging of skin	☐	☐	
Color	☐	☐	
Dimpling	☐	☐	
Puckering	☐	☐	
Shape	☐	☐	
Size	☐	☐	
Swelling	☐	☐	
Pain	☐	☐	1 2 3 4 5 6 7 8 9 10
Soreness	☐	☐	1 2 3 4 5 6 7 8 9 10

Nipple

Position	☐	☐
Ex: position change: Inward instead of pushing outward		
Redness	☐	☐
Ex: Position change: Inward instead of pushing outward		
Fluid	☐	☐
Ex: blood, milky, yellow fluid, or watery		

Position	☐	☐
Ex: position change: Inward instead of pushing outward		
Redness	☐	☐
Ex: Position change: Inward instead of pushing outward		
Fluid	☐	☐
Ex: blood, milky, yellow fluid, or watery		

Lump

Bulging of skin	☐	☐
Color	☐	☐
Dimpling	☐	☐

Bulging of skin	☐	☐
Color	☐	☐
Dimpling	☐	☐

Next steps: Notified Dr. ☐   Dr's Appointment ☐

Label lump, pain, and/or create your own label

USE L = LUMP   **USE P = PAIN**

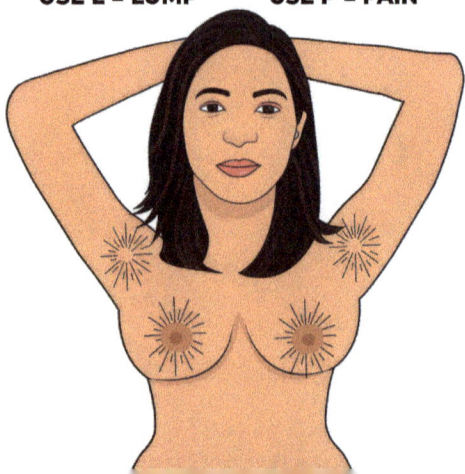

HAPPY SCALE

AM	PM
1	1
2	2
3	3
4	4
5	5
6	6
7	7
8	8
9	9
10	10

NOTES / DOODLES

Get to know your breasts

DATE ————————————————— TIME —————————————————

Left	Right
Do you notice any changes?	**Do you notice any changes?**

Overall Breast Health

	Yes	No	If yes, what is different?
Bulging of skin	☐	☐	
Color	☐	☐	
Dimpling	☐	☐	
Puckering	☐	☐	
Shape	☐	☐	
Size	☐	☐	
Swelling	☐	☐	
Pain	☐	☐	1 2 3 4 5 6 7 8 9 10
Soreness	☐	☐	1 2 3 4 5 6 7 8 9 10

	Yes	No	If yes, what is different?
Bulging of skin	☐	☐	
Color	☐	☐	
Dimpling	☐	☐	
Puckering	☐	☐	
Shape	☐	☐	
Size	☐	☐	
Swelling	☐	☐	
Pain	☐	☐	1 2 3 4 5 6 7 8 9 10
Soreness	☐	☐	1 2 3 4 5 6 7 8 9 10

Nipple

Position ☐ ☐
Ex: position change: Inward instead of pushing outward

Redness ☐ ☐
Ex: Position change: Inward instead of pushing outward

Fluid ☐ ☐
Ex: blood, milky, yellow fluid, or watery

Position ☐ ☐
Ex: position change: Inward instead of pushing outward

Redness ☐ ☐
Ex: Position change: Inward instead of pushing outward

Fluid ☐ ☐
Ex: blood, milky, yellow fluid, or watery

Lump

Bulging of skin ☐ ☐

Color ☐ ☐

Dimpling ☐ ☐

Bulging of skin ☐ ☐

Color ☐ ☐

Dimpling ☐ ☐

Next steps: Notified Dr. ☐   Dr's Appointment ☐

Label Lump, pain, and/or create your own Label
USE L = LUMP   **USE P = PAIN**

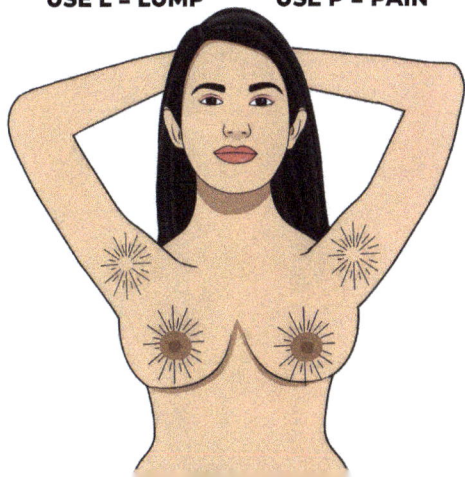

HAPPY SCALE

AM	PM
1	1
2	2
3	3
4	4
5	5
6	6
7	7
8	8
9	9
10	10

NOTES / DOODLES

81

Get to know your breasts

DATE _____   TIME _____

Left	Right
Do you notice any changes?	**Do you notice any changes?**

Overall Breast Health

	Yes	No	If yes, what is different?
Bulging of skin	☐	☐	
Color	☐	☐	
Dimpling	☐	☐	
Puckering	☐	☐	
Shape	☐	☐	
Size	☐	☐	
Swelling	☐	☐	
Pain	☐	☐	1 2 3 4 5 6 7 8 9 10
Soreness	☐	☐	1 2 3 4 5 6 7 8 9 10

	Yes	No	If yes, what is different?
Bulging of skin	☐	☐	
Color	☐	☐	
Dimpling	☐	☐	
Puckering	☐	☐	
Shape	☐	☐	
Size	☐	☐	
Swelling	☐	☐	
Pain	☐	☐	1 2 3 4 5 6 7 8 9 10
Soreness	☐	☐	1 2 3 4 5 6 7 8 9 10

Nipple

Position ☐ ☐		
Ex: position change: Inward instead of pushing outward		
Redness ☐ ☐		
Ex: Position change: Inward instead of pushing outward		
Fluid ☐ ☐		
Ex: blood, milky, yellow fluid, or watery		

Position ☐ ☐		
Ex: position change: Inward instead of pushing outward		
Redness ☐ ☐		
Ex: Position change: Inward instead of pushing outward		
Fluid ☐ ☐		
Ex: blood, milky, yellow fluid, or watery		

Lump

Bulging of skin ☐ ☐		
Color ☐ ☐		
Dimpling ☐ ☐		

Bulging of skin ☐ ☐		
Color ☐ ☐		
Dimpling ☐ ☐		

Next steps: Notified Dr. ☐   Dr's Appointment ☐

Label lump, pain, and/or create your own label

USE L = LUMP   USE P = PAIN

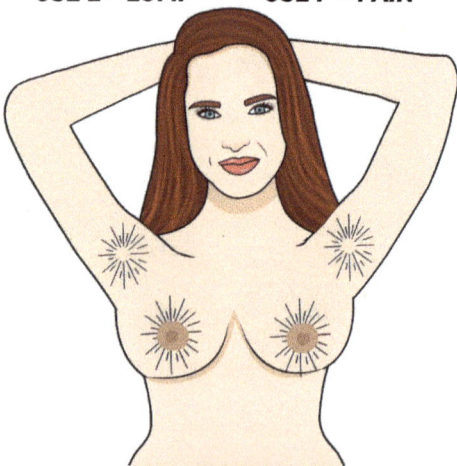

HAPPY SCALE

AM	PM
1	1
2	2
3	3
4	4
5	5
6	6
7	7
8	8
9	9
10	10

NOTES / DOODLES

Get to know your breasts

DATE _____ TIME _____

Left	Right
Do you notice any changes?	**Do you notice any changes?**

Overall Breast Health

	Yes	No	If yes, what is different?
Bulging of skin	☐	☐	
Color	☐	☐	
Dimpling	☐	☐	
Puckering	☐	☐	
Shape	☐	☐	
Size	☐	☐	
Swelling	☐	☐	
Pain	☐	☐	1 2 3 4 5 6 7 8 9 10
Soreness	☐	☐	1 2 3 4 5 6 7 8 9 10

	Yes	No	If yes, what is different?
Bulging of skin	☐	☐	
Color	☐	☐	
Dimpling	☐	☐	
Puckering	☐	☐	
Shape	☐	☐	
Size	☐	☐	
Swelling	☐	☐	
Pain	☐	☐	1 2 3 4 5 6 7 8 9 10
Soreness	☐	☐	1 2 3 4 5 6 7 8 9 10

Nipple

Position	☐	☐
Ex: position change: Inward instead of pushing outward		
Redness	☐	☐
Ex: Position change: Inward instead of pushing outward		
Fluid	☐	☐
Ex: blood, milky, yellow fluid, or watery		

Position	☐	☐
Ex: position change: Inward instead of pushing outward		
Redness	☐	☐
Ex: Position change: Inward instead of pushing outward		
Fluid	☐	☐
Ex: blood, milky, yellow fluid, or watery		

Lump

Bulging of skin	☐	☐
Color	☐	☐
Dimpling	☐	☐

Bulging of skin	☐	☐
Color	☐	☐
Dimpling	☐	☐

Next steps: Notified Dr. ☐   Dr's Appointment ☐

Label lump, pain, and/or create your own label

USE L = LUMP   **USE P = PAIN**

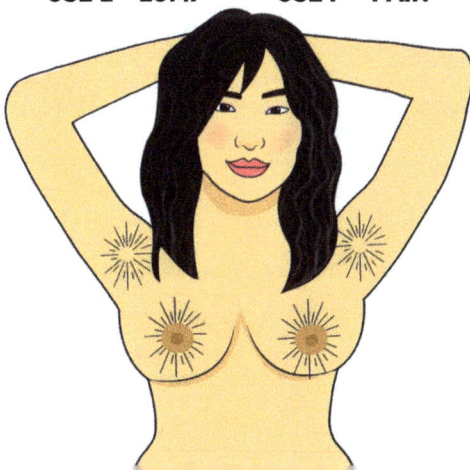

HAPPY SCALE

AM	PM
1	1
2	2
3	3
4	4
5	5
6	6
7	7
8	8
9	9
10	10

NOTES / DOODLES

Get to know your breasts

DATE _____   TIME _____

Left	Right
Do you notice any changes?	**Do you notice any changes?**

Overall Breast Health

	Yes	No	If yes, what is different?
Bulging of skin	☐	☐	
Color	☐	☐	
Dimpling	☐	☐	
Puckering	☐	☐	
Shape	☐	☐	
Size	☐	☐	
Swelling	☐	☐	
Pain	☐	☐	1 2 3 4 5 6 7 8 9 10
Soreness	☐	☐	1 2 3 4 5 6 7 8 9 10

	Yes	No	If yes, what is different?
Bulging of skin	☐	☐	
Color	☐	☐	
Dimpling	☐	☐	
Puckering	☐	☐	
Shape	☐	☐	
Size	☐	☐	
Swelling	☐	☐	
Pain	☐	☐	1 2 3 4 5 6 7 8 9 10
Soreness	☐	☐	1 2 3 4 5 6 7 8 9 10

Nipple

Position ☐ ☐
Ex: position change: Inward instead of pushing outward

Redness ☐ ☐
Ex: Position change: Inward instead of pushing outward

Fluid ☐ ☐
Ex: blood, milky, yellow fluid, or watery

Position ☐ ☐
Ex: position change: Inward instead of pushing outward

Redness ☐ ☐
Ex: Position change: Inward instead of pushing outward

Fluid ☐ ☐
Ex: blood, milky, yellow fluid, or watery

Lump

Bulging of skin	☐ ☐
Color	☐ ☐
Dimpling	☐ ☐

Bulging of skin	☐ ☐
Color	☐ ☐
Dimpling	☐ ☐

Next steps: Notified Dr. ☐   Dr's Appointment ☐

Label lump, pain, and/or create your own label

USE L = LUMP   USE P = PAIN

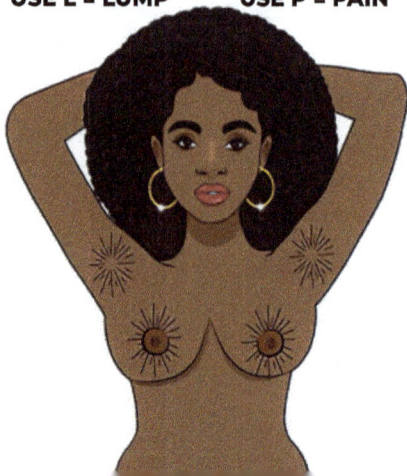

HAPPY SCALE

AM	PM
1	1
2	2
3	3
4	4
5	5
6	6
7	7
8	8
9	9
10	10

NOTES / DOODLES

Get to know your breasts

DATE _____ TIME _____

Left	Right
Do you notice any changes?	**Do you notice any changes?**

Overall Breast Health

	Yes	No	If yes, what is different?		Yes	No	If yes, what is different?
Bulging of skin	☐	☐		**Bulging of skin**	☐	☐	
Color	☐	☐		**Color**	☐	☐	
Dimpling	☐	☐		**Dimpling**	☐	☐	
Puckering	☐	☐		**Puckering**	☐	☐	
Shape	☐	☐		**Shape**	☐	☐	
Size	☐	☐		**Size**	☐	☐	
Swelling	☐	☐		**Swelling**	☐	☐	
Pain	☐	☐	1 2 3 4 5 6 7 8 9 10	**Pain**	☐	☐	1 2 3 4 5 6 7 8 9 10
Soreness	☐	☐	1 2 3 4 5 6 7 8 9 10	**Soreness**	☐	☐	1 2 3 4 5 6 7 8 9 10

Nipple

	Yes	No			Yes	No
Position	☐	☐		**Position**	☐	☐
Ex: position change: Inward instead of pushing outward				*Ex: position change: Inward instead of pushing outward*		
Redness	☐	☐		**Redness**	☐	☐
Ex: Position change: Inward instead of pushing outward				*Ex: Position change: Inward instead of pushing outward*		
Fluid	☐	☐		**Fluid**	☐	☐
Ex: blood, milky, yellow fluid, or watery				*Ex: blood, milky, yellow fluid, or watery*		

Lump

	Yes	No			Yes	No
Bulging of skin	☐	☐		**Bulging of skin**	☐	☐
Color	☐	☐		**Color**	☐	☐
Dimpling	☐	☐		**Dimpling**	☐	☐

Next steps: Notified Dr. ☐   Dr's Appointment ☐

Label Lump, pain, and/or create your own label

USE L = LUMP   **USE P = PAIN**

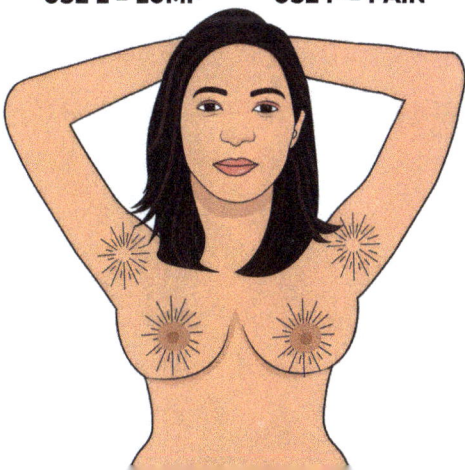

HAPPY SCALE

AM	PM
1	1
2	2
3	3
4	4
5	5
6	6
7	7
8	8
9	9
10	10

NOTES / DOODLES

Get to know your breasts

DATE _____   TIME _____

Left
Do you notice any changes?

Right
Do you notice any changes?

Overall Breast Health

	Yes	No	If yes, what is different?
Bulging of skin	☐	☐	
Color	☐	☐	
Dimpling	☐	☐	
Puckering	☐	☐	
Shape	☐	☐	
Size	☐	☐	
Swelling	☐	☐	
Pain	☐	☐	1 2 3 4 5 6 7 8 9 10
Soreness	☐	☐	1 2 3 4 5 6 7 8 9 10

	Yes	No	If yes, what is different?
Bulging of skin	☐	☐	
Color	☐	☐	
Dimpling	☐	☐	
Puckering	☐	☐	
Shape	☐	☐	
Size	☐	☐	
Swelling	☐	☐	
Pain	☐	☐	1 2 3 4 5 6 7 8 9 10
Soreness	☐	☐	1 2 3 4 5 6 7 8 9 10

Nipple

Position	☐	☐

Ex: position change: Inward instead of pushing outward

Redness	☐	☐

Ex: Position change: Inward instead of pushing outward

Fluid	☐	☐

Ex: blood, milky, yellow fluid, or watery

Position	☐	☐

Ex: position change: Inward instead of pushing outward

Redness	☐	☐

Ex: Position change: Inward instead of pushing outward

Fluid	☐	☐

Ex: blood, milky, yellow fluid, or watery

Lump

Bulging of skin	☐	☐
Color	☐	☐
Dimpling	☐	☐

Bulging of skin	☐	☐
Color	☐	☐
Dimpling	☐	☐

Next steps: Notified Dr. ☐   Dr's Appointment ☐

Label lump, pain, and/or create your own label

USE L = LUMP   USE P = PAIN

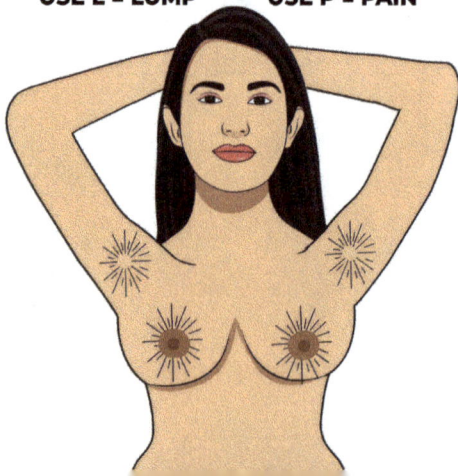

HAPPY SCALE

AM	PM
1	1
2	2
3	3
4	4
5	5
6	6
7	7
8	8
9	9
10	10

NOTES / DOODLES

Get to know your breasts

DATE _____ **TIME** _____

Left
Do you notice any changes?

Right
Do you notice any changes?

Overall Breast Health

	Yes	No	If yes, what is different?
Bulging of skin	☐	☐	
Color	☐	☐	
Dimpling	☐	☐	
Puckering	☐	☐	
Shape	☐	☐	
Size	☐	☐	
Swelling	☐	☐	
Pain	☐	☐	1 2 3 4 5 6 7 8 9 10
Soreness	☐	☐	1 2 3 4 5 6 7 8 9 10

	Yes	No	If yes, what is different?
Bulging of skin	☐	☐	
Color	☐	☐	
Dimpling	☐	☐	
Puckering	☐	☐	
Shape	☐	☐	
Size	☐	☐	
Swelling	☐	☐	
Pain	☐	☐	1 2 3 4 5 6 7 8 9 10
Soreness	☐	☐	1 2 3 4 5 6 7 8 9 10

Nipple

Position	☐	☐

Ex: position change: Inward instead of pushing outward

Redness	☐	☐

Ex: Position change: Inward instead of pushing outward

Fluid	☐	☐

Ex: blood, milky, yellow fluid, or watery

Position	☐	☐

Ex: position change: Inward instead of pushing outward

Redness	☐	☐

Ex: Position change: Inward instead of pushing outward

Fluid	☐	☐

Ex: blood, milky, yellow fluid, or watery

Lump

Bulging of skin	☐	☐
Color	☐	☐
Dimpling	☐	☐

Bulging of skin	☐	☐
Color	☐	☐
Dimpling	☐	☐

Next steps: Notified Dr. ☐   Dr's Appointment ☐

Label Lump, pain, and/or create your own Label

USE L = LUMP   **USE P = PAIN**

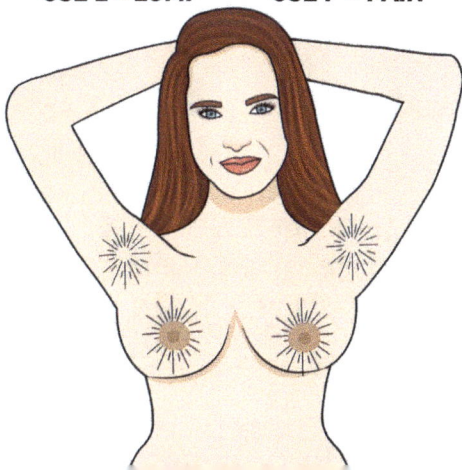

HAPPY SCALE

AM	PM
1	1
2	2
3	3
4	4
5	5
6	6
7	7
8	8
9	9
10	10

NOTES / DOODLES

Get to know your breasts

DATE _____   **TIME** _____

Left
Do you notice any changes?

Right
Do you notice any changes?

Overall Breast Health

	Yes	No	If yes, what is different?
Bulging of skin	☐	☐	
Color	☐	☐	
Dimpling	☐	☐	
Puckering	☐	☐	
Shape	☐	☐	
Size	☐	☐	
Swelling	☐	☐	
Pain	☐	☐	1 2 3 4 5 6 7 8 9 10
Soreness	☐	☐	1 2 3 4 5 6 7 8 9 10

	Yes	No	If yes, what is different?
Bulging of skin	☐	☐	
Color	☐	☐	
Dimpling	☐	☐	
Puckering	☐	☐	
Shape	☐	☐	
Size	☐	☐	
Swelling	☐	☐	
Pain	☐	☐	1 2 3 4 5 6 7 8 9 10
Soreness	☐	☐	1 2 3 4 5 6 7 8 9 10

Nipple

Position	☐	☐	

Ex: position change: Inward instead of pushing outward

Redness	☐	☐	

Ex: Position change: Inward instead of pushing outward

Fluid	☐	☐	

Ex: blood, milky, yellow fluid, or watery

Position	☐	☐	

Ex: position change: Inward instead of pushing outward

Redness	☐	☐	

Ex: Position change: Inward instead of pushing outward

Fluid	☐	☐	

Ex: blood, milky, yellow fluid, or watery

Lump

Bulging of skin	☐ ☐
Color	☐ ☐
Dimpling	☐ ☐

Bulging of skin	☐ ☐
Color	☐ ☐
Dimpling	☐ ☐

Next steps: Notified Dr. ☐   Dr's Appointment ☐

Label lump, pain, and/or create your own label

USE L = LUMP   **USE P = PAIN**

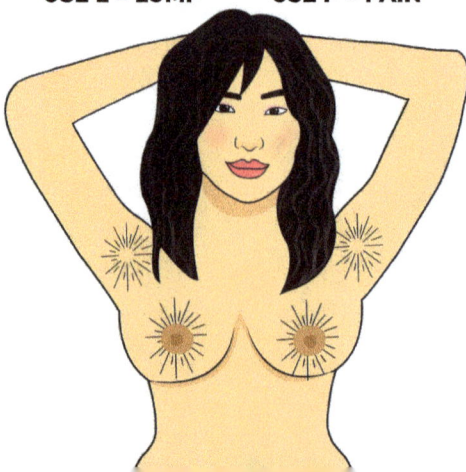

HAPPY SCALE

AM	PM
1	1
2	2
3	3
4	4
5	5
6	6
7	7
8	8
9	9
10	10

NOTES / DOODLES

HOW AM I FEELING TODAY?

☐ ☐ ☐ ☐ ☐ ☐ ☐ ☐ ☐ ☐

NOT GREAT   INCREDIBLE

Doctor's name & info

REASON FOR VISIT

_____
_____
_____
_____
_____
_____

INSTRUCTIONS GUIDE

_____
_____
_____
_____

RESULTS

_____
_____
_____
_____
_____

EMOTIONAL WHEEL

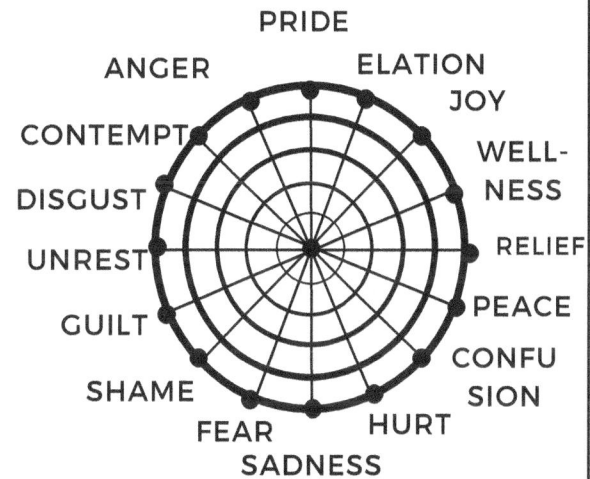

PRIDE

ANGER   ELATION

     JOY

CONTEMPT   WELL-NESS

DISGUST

UNREST   RELIEF

GUILT   PEACE

SHAME   CONFUSION

FEAR   HURT

SADNESS

NEXT STEPS

_____
_____
_____
_____
_____

Things to celebrate......

_____
_____
_____
_____
_____

NEXT APPOINTMENT DATE & TIME

HOW AM I FEELING TODAY?

☐ ☐ ☐ ☐ ☐ ☐ ☐ ☐ ☐ ☐

NOT GREAT   INCREDIBLE

Doctor's name & info

REASON FOR VISIT

_____
_____
_____
_____
_____

INSTRUCTIONS GUIDE

_____
_____
_____

NEXT STEPS

_____
_____
_____
_____
_____

RESULTS

_____
_____
_____
_____
_____

EMOTIONAL WHEEL

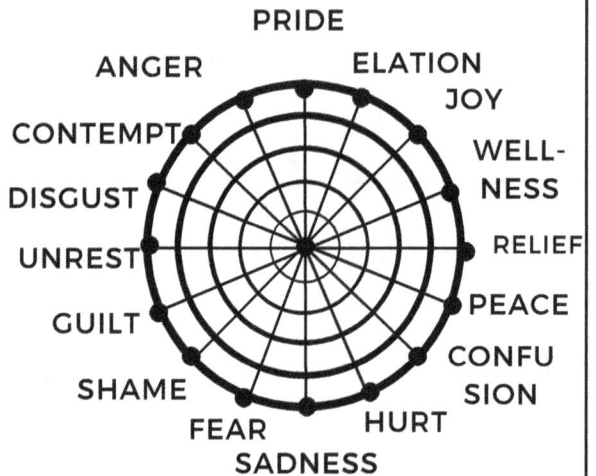

PRIDE
ANGER   ELATION
                JOY
CONTEMPT
                WELL-
DISGUST   NESS
UNREST   RELIEF
GUILT   PEACE
              CONFU
SHAME   SION
  FEAR   HURT
  SADNESS

Things to celebrate......

_____
_____
_____
_____
_____

NEXT APPOINTMENT DATE & TIME

Check in

Doctor's APPOINTMENT   DATE _____

HOW AM I FEELING TODAY?

☐ ☐ ☐ ☐ ☐ ☐ ☐ ☐ ☐ ☐

NOT GREAT   INCREDIBLE

Doctor's name & info

REASON FOR VISIT

_____

_____

_____

_____

_____

_____

INSTRUCTIONS GUIDE

_____

_____

_____

RESULTS

_____

_____

_____

_____

_____

EMOTIONAL WHEEL

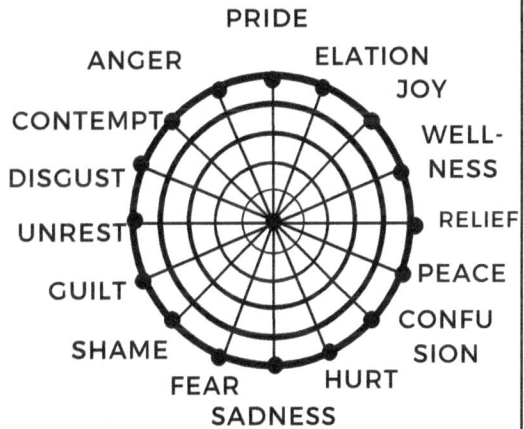

PRIDE

ANGER   ELATION

JOY

CONTEMPT   WELL-NESS

DISGUST   RELIEF

UNREST   PEACE

GUILT   CONFU SION

SHAME   HURT

FEAR   SADNESS

NEXT STEPS

_____

_____

_____

_____

_____

Things to celebrate ......

_____

_____

_____

_____

NEXT APPOINTMENT DATE & TIME

Check in

Doctor's APPOINTMENT   DATE _____

HOW AM I FEELING TODAY?

☐ ☐ ☐ ☐ ☐ ☐ ☐ ☐ ☐ ☐

NOT GREAT   INCREDIBLE

Doctor's name & info

REASON FOR VISIT

_____

_____

_____

_____

_____

INSTRUCTIONS GUIDE

_____

_____

_____

_____

NEXT STEPS

_____

_____

_____

_____

_____

RESULTS

_____

_____

_____

_____

_____

EMOTIONAL WHEEL

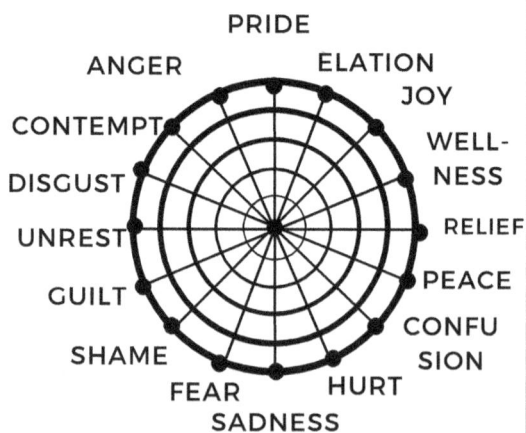

PRIDE

ANGER   ELATION

JOY

CONTEMPT   WELL-
                  NESS

DISGUST

                  RELIEF

UNREST

                  PEACE

GUILT   CONFU
               SION

SHAME

     FEAR   HURT

     SADNESS

Things to celebrate .....

_____

_____

_____

_____

_____

NEXT APPOINTMENT DATE & TIME

Check in

Doctor's APPOINTMENT   DATE _____

HOW AM I FEELING TODAY?

☐ ☐ ☐ ☐ ☐ ☐ ☐ ☐ ☐ ☐

NOT GREAT   INCREDIBLE

Doctor's name & info

REASON FOR VISIT

_____

_____

_____

_____

_____

INSTRUCTIONS GUIDE

_____

_____

_____

_____

RESULTS

_____

_____

_____

_____

_____

_____

EMOTIONAL WHEEL

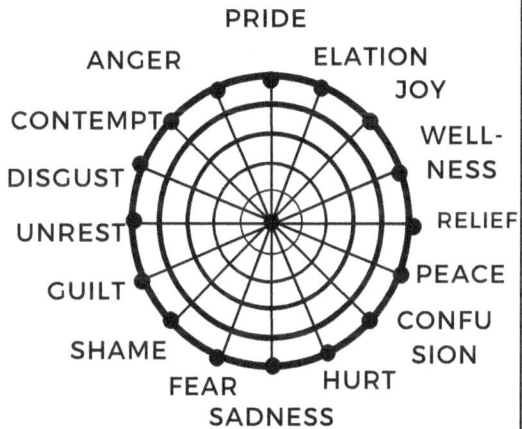

PRIDE
ANGER   ELATION
JOY
CONTEMPT   WELL-NESS
DISGUST
UNREST   RELIEF
GUILT   PEACE
CONFU SION
SHAME   HURT
FEAR
SADNESS

NEXT STEPS

_____

_____

_____

_____

_____

Things to celebrate ......

_____

_____

_____

_____

NEXT APPOINTMENT DATE & TIME

Check in

Doctor's APPOINTMENT   DATE _____

HOW AM I FEELING TODAY?

☐ ☐ ☐ ☐ ☐ ☐ ☐ ☐ ☐ ☐

NOT GREAT   INCREDIBLE

Doctor's name & info

REASON FOR VISIT

_____
_____
_____
_____
_____

INSTRUCTIONS GUIDE

_____
_____
_____
_____

RESULTS

_____
_____
_____
_____
_____

EMOTIONAL WHEEL

PRIDE

ANGER   ELATION
                              JOY
CONTEMPT
                          WELL-
DISGUST   NESS

UNREST   RELIEF

GUILT   PEACE

SHAME   CONFU
                            SION
        FEAR   HURT
        SADNESS

NEXT STEPS

_____
_____
_____
_____
_____

Things to celebrate ......

_____
_____
_____
_____
_____

NEXT APPOINTMENT DATE & TIME

Check in

Doctor's APPOINTMENT   DATE _____

HOW AM I FEELING TODAY?

☐ ☐ ☐ ☐ ☐ ☐ ☐ ☐ ☐ ☐

NOT GREAT   INCREDIBLE

Doctor's name & info

REASON FOR VISIT

_____

_____

_____

_____

_____

INSTRUCTIONS GUIDE

_____

_____

_____

_____

NEXT STEPS

_____

_____

_____

_____

_____

RESULTS

_____

_____

_____

_____

_____

EMOTIONAL WHEEL

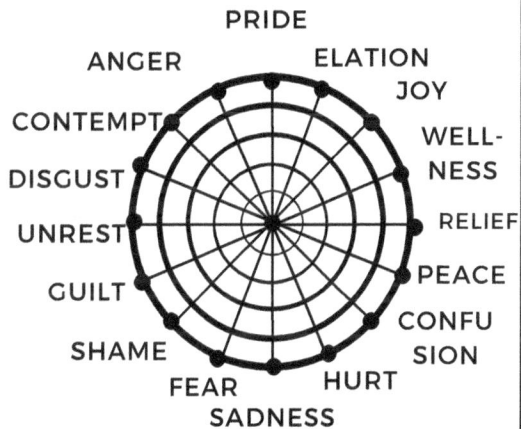

PRIDE

ANGER   ELATION

JOY

CONTEMPT

WELL-NESS

DISGUST

RELIEF

UNREST

PEACE

GUILT   CONFU SION

SHAME

FEAR   HURT

SADNESS

Things to celebrate......

_____

_____

_____

_____

_____

NEXT APPOINTMENT DATE & TIME

Check in

Doctor's APPOINTMENT   DATE _____

HOW AM I FEELING TODAY?

☐ ☐ ☐ ☐ ☐ ☐ ☐ ☐ ☐ ☐

NOT GREAT   INCREDIBLE

Doctor's name &
info

REASON FOR VISIT

_____
_____
_____
_____
_____
_____

INSTRUCTIONS GUIDE

_____
_____
_____
_____

RESULTS

_____
_____
_____
_____
_____
_____

EMOTIONAL WHEEL

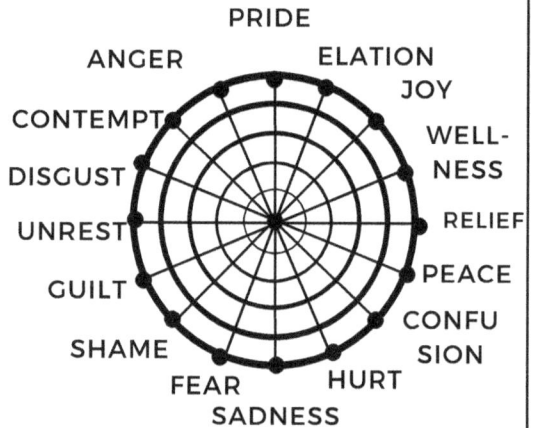

PRIDE
ANGER   ELATION
JOY
CONTEMPT
WELL-
NESS
DISGUST
UNREST   RELIEF
GUILT   PEACE
SHAME   CONFU
SION
FEAR   HURT
SADNESS

NEXT STEPS

_____
_____
_____
_____
_____

Things to celebrate ......

_____
_____
_____
_____
_____

NEXT APPOINTMENT DATE & TIME

Check in

Doctor's APPOINTMENT   DATE _____

HOW AM I FEELING TODAY?

☐ ☐ ☐ ☐ ☐ ☐ ☐ ☐ ☐ ☐

NOT GREAT   INCREDIBLE

Doctor's name & info

RESULTS

_____
_____
_____
_____
_____

REASON FOR VISIT

_____
_____
_____
_____
_____

INSTRUCTIONS GUIDE

_____
_____
_____
_____

EMOTIONAL WHEEL

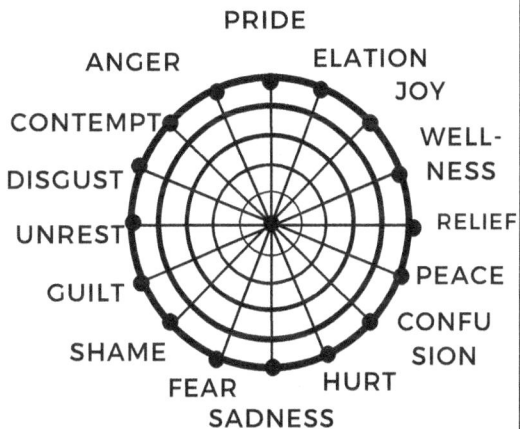

PRIDE
ANGER   ELATION
                JOY
CONTEMPT   WELL-
                NESS
DISGUST
UNREST   RELIEF
GUILT   PEACE
                CONFU
SHAME   SION
     FEAR   HURT
     SADNESS

NEXT STEPS

_____
_____
_____
_____
_____

Things to celebrate......

_____
_____
_____
_____

NEXT APPOINTMENT DATE & TIME

Check in

Doctor's APPOINTMENT   DATE _____

HOW AM I FEELING TODAY?

☐ ☐ ☐ ☐ ☐ ☐ ☐ ☐ ☐

NOT GREAT   INCREDIBLE

Doctor's name & info

REASON FOR VISIT

_____
_____
_____
_____
_____
_____

INSTRUCTIONS GUIDE

_____
_____
_____
_____

RESULTS

_____
_____
_____
_____
_____

EMOTIONAL WHEEL

PRIDE
ANGER   ELATION
                        JOY
CONTEMPT
                    WELL-
                    NESS
DISGUST
UNREST   RELIEF
GUILT   PEACE
                    CONFU
SHAME   SION
        FEAR   HURT
        SADNESS

NEXT STEPS

_____
_____
_____
_____
_____

Things to celebrate......

_____
_____
_____
_____
_____

NEXT APPOINTMENT DATE & TIME

Check in

Doctor's APPOINTMENT

DATE _____

HOW AM I FEELING TODAY?

☐ ☐ ☐ ☐ ☐ ☐ ☐ ☐ ☐ ☐

NOT GREAT   INCREDIBLE

Doctor's name &
info

REASON FOR VISIT

_____

_____

_____

_____

_____

_____

INSTRUCTIONS GUIDE

_____

_____

_____

_____

NEXT STEPS

_____

_____

_____

_____

_____

RESULTS

_____

_____

_____

_____

_____

EMOTIONAL WHEEL

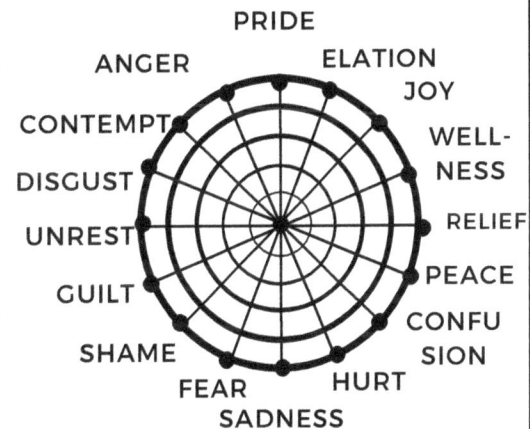

PRIDE

ANGER

ELATION

JOY

CONTEMPT

WELL-NESS

DISGUST

RELIEF

UNREST

PEACE

GUILT

CONFU-SION

SHAME

HURT

FEAR

SADNESS

Things to celebrate ......

_____

_____

_____

_____

_____

NEXT APPOINTMENT DATE & TIME

Check in

Doctor's APPOINTMENT   DATE _____

HOW AM I FEELING TODAY?

☐ ☐ ☐ ☐ ☐ ☐ ☐ ☐ ☐ ☐

NOT GREAT   INCREDIBLE

*Doctor's name &
info*

REASON FOR VISIT

_____
_____
_____
_____
_____

INSTRUCTIONS GUIDE

_____
_____
_____
_____

NEXT STEPS

_____
_____
_____
_____
_____

RESULTS

_____
_____
_____
_____
_____

EMOTIONAL WHEEL

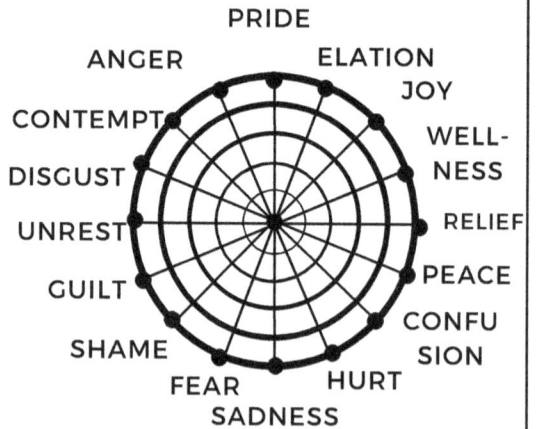

PRIDE
ANGER   ELATION
              JOY
CONTEMPT
              WELL-
DISGUST   NESS
UNREST   RELIEF
GUILT   PEACE
              CONFU
SHAME   SION
   FEAR   HURT
   SADNESS

Things to celebrate ......

_____
_____
_____
_____

NEXT APPOINTMENT DATE & TIME

Check in

Doctor's APPOINTMENT   DATE _____

HOW AM I FEELING TODAY?

☐ ☐ ☐ ☐ ☐ ☐ ☐ ☐ ☐ ☐

NOT GREAT   INCREDIBLE

Doctor's name &
info

REASON FOR VISIT

_____

_____

_____

_____

_____

INSTRUCTIONS GUIDE

_____

_____

_____

_____

RESULTS

_____

_____

_____

_____

_____

_____

EMOTIONAL WHEEL

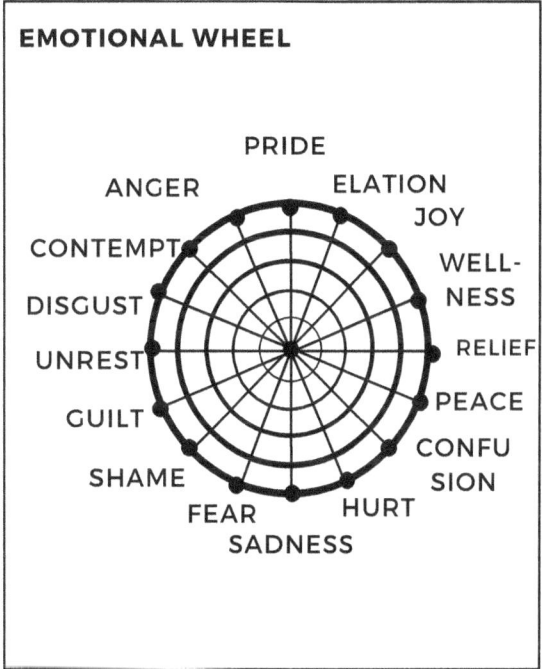

PRIDE

ANGER   ELATION

JOY

CONTEMPT

WELL-
NESS

DISGUST

RELIEF

UNREST

PEACE

GUILT   CONFU
SION

SHAME

HURT

FEAR

SADNESS

NEXT STEPS

_____

_____

_____

_____

_____

Things to celebrate......

_____

_____

_____

_____

_____

NEXT APPOINTMENT DATE & TIME

Check in

Doctor's APPOINTMENT   DATE _____

HOW AM I FEELING TODAY?

☐ ☐ ☐ ☐ ☐ ☐ ☐ ☐ ☐ ☐

NOT GREAT   INCREDIBLE

Doctor's name & info

REASON FOR VISIT

_____

_____

_____

_____

_____

INSTRUCTIONS GUIDE

_____

_____

_____

_____

RESULTS

_____

_____

_____

_____

_____

EMOTIONAL WHEEL

PRIDE

ANGER   ELATION

                              JOY

CONTEMPT

                         WELL-
DISGUST   NESS

UNREST   RELIEF

GUILT   PEACE

                         CONFU
SHAME   SION

        FEAR   HURT
        SADNESS

NEXT STEPS

_____

_____

_____

_____

Things to celebrate......

_____

_____

_____

_____

NEXT APPOINTMENT DATE & TIME

Check in

Doctor's APPOINTMENT   DATE _____

HOW AM I FEELING TODAY?

☐ ☐ ☐ ☐ ☐ ☐ ☐ ☐ ☐ ☐

NOT GREAT   INCREDIBLE

Doctor's name &
info

REASON FOR VISIT

_____
_____
_____
_____
_____

INSTRUCTIONS GUIDE

_____
_____
_____

RESULTS

_____
_____
_____
_____
_____

EMOTIONAL WHEEL

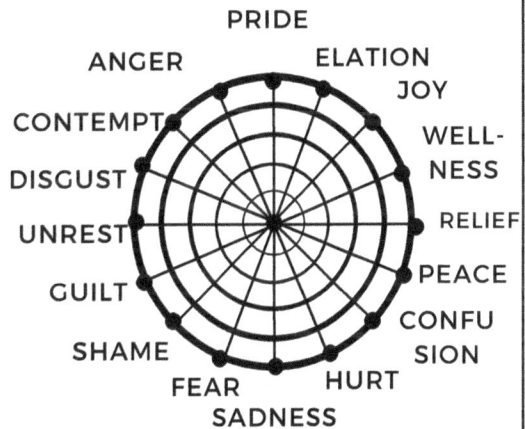

PRIDE

ANGER   ELATION
                      JOY

CONTEMPT   WELL-
                          NESS

DISGUST

UNREST   RELIEF

GUILT   PEACE

SHAME   CONFU
                      SION

FEAR   HURT
SADNESS

NEXT STEPS

_____
_____
_____
_____
_____

Things to celebrate......

_____
_____
_____
_____

NEXT APPOINTMENT DATE & TIME

Check in

Doctor's APPOINTMENT   DATE _____

HOW AM I FEELING TODAY?

☐ ☐ ☐ ☐ ☐ ☐ ☐ ☐ ☐ ☐

NOT GREAT   INCREDIBLE

Doctor's name & info

REASON FOR VISIT

_____
_____
_____
_____
_____

INSTRUCTIONS GUIDE

_____
_____
_____
_____

RESULTS

_____
_____
_____
_____
_____

EMOTIONAL WHEEL

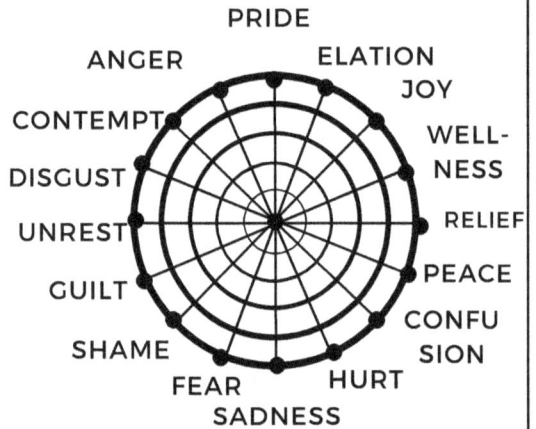

PRIDE
ANGER   ELATION
                        JOY
CONTEMPT
                   WELL-
DISGUST   NESS
UNREST   RELIEF
GUILT   PEACE
                   CONFU
SHAME   SION
       FEAR   HURT
       SADNESS

NEXT STEPS

_____
_____
_____
_____
_____

Things to celebrate ......

_____
_____
_____
_____
_____

NEXT APPOINTMENT DATE & TIME

Check in

Doctor's APPOINTMENT   DATE _____

HOW AM I FEELING TODAY?

☐ ☐ ☐ ☐ ☐ ☐ ☐ ☐ ☐ ☐

NOT GREAT   INCREDIBLE

Doctor's name & info

REASON FOR VISIT

_____
_____
_____
_____
_____

INSTRUCTIONS GUIDE

_____
_____
_____
_____

RESULTS

_____
_____
_____
_____
_____

EMOTIONAL WHEEL

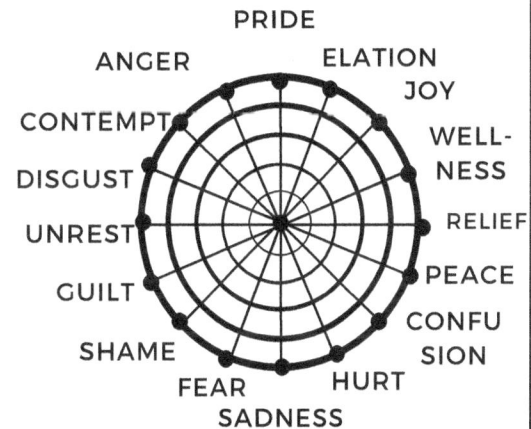

PRIDE
ANGER   ELATION
                JOY
CONTEMPT
                 WELL-
DISGUST   NESS
                RELIEF
UNREST
                PEACE
GUILT   CONFU
                SION
SHAME
      FEAR   HURT
      SADNESS

NEXT STEPS

_____
_____
_____
_____
_____

Things to celebrate......

_____
_____
_____
_____

NEXT APPOINTMENT DATE & TIME

Check in

Doctor's APPOINTMENT   DATE _____

HOW AM I FEELING TODAY?

☐ ☐ ☐ ☐ ☐ ☐ ☐ ☐ ☐ ☐

NOT GREAT   INCREDIBLE

Doctor's name &
info

REASON FOR VISIT

_____
_____
_____
_____
_____

INSTRUCTIONS GUIDE

_____
_____
_____
_____

RESULTS

_____
_____
_____
_____
_____

EMOTIONAL WHEEL

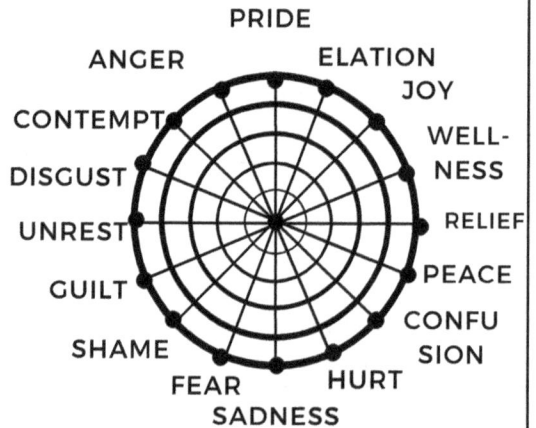

PRIDE
ANGER   ELATION
                JOY
CONTEMPT
                WELL-
DISGUST   NESS
UNREST   RELIEF
GUILT   PEACE
                CONFU
SHAME   SION
      FEAR   HURT
      SADNESS

NEXT STEPS

_____
_____
_____
_____
_____

Things to celebrate......

_____
_____
_____
_____
_____

NEXT APPOINTMENT DATE & TIME

Check in

Doctor's **APPOINTMENT**   DATE _____

HOW AM I FEELING TODAY?

☐ ☐ ☐ ☐ ☐ ☐ ☐ ☐ ☐ ☐

NOT GREAT   INCREDIBLE

Doctor's name & info

REASON FOR VISIT

_____

_____

_____

_____

_____

INSTRUCTIONS GUIDE

_____

_____

_____

_____

RESULTS

_____

_____

_____

_____

_____

EMOTIONAL WHEEL

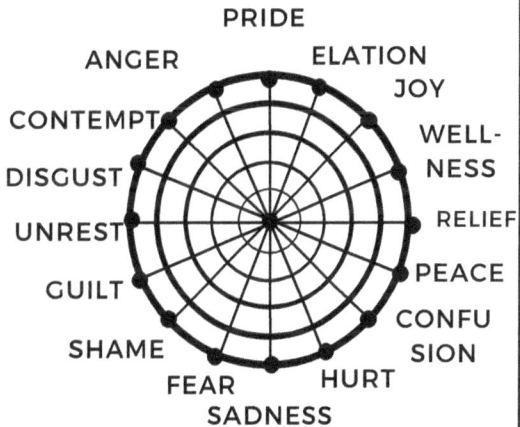

PRIDE

ANGER   ELATION

JOY

CONTEMPT   WELL-
NESS

DISGUST

RELIEF

UNREST

PEACE

GUILT   CONFU
SION

SHAME

FEAR   HURT

SADNESS

NEXT STEPS

_____

_____

_____

_____

_____

Things to celebrate ......

_____

_____

_____

_____

NEXT APPOINTMENT DATE & TIME

Check in

Doctor's APPOINTMENT   DATE _____

HOW AM I FEELING TODAY?

☐ ☐ ☐ ☐ ☐ ☐ ☐ ☐ ☐ ☐

NOT GREAT   INCREDIBLE

Doctor's name & info

REASON FOR VISIT

_____
_____
_____
_____
_____
_____

INSTRUCTIONS GUIDE

_____
_____
_____
_____

RESULTS

_____
_____
_____
_____
_____

EMOTIONAL WHEEL

PRIDE
ANGER   ELATION
                JOY
CONTEMPT
                WELL-
DISGUST   NESS
UNREST   RELIEF
GUILT   PEACE
                CONFU
SHAME   SION
     FEAR   HURT
     SADNESS

NEXT STEPS

_____
_____
_____
_____
_____

Things to celebrate......

_____
_____
_____
_____

NEXT APPOINTMENT DATE & TIME

Check in

Doctor's APPOINTMENT DATE _____

HOW AM I FEELING TODAY?

☐ ☐ ☐ ☐ ☐ ☐ ☐ ☐ ☐

NOT GREAT   INCREDIBLE

Doctor's name & info

REASON FOR VISIT

_____

_____

_____

_____

_____

INSTRUCTIONS GUIDE

_____

_____

_____

_____

RESULTS

_____

_____

_____

_____

_____

EMOTIONAL WHEEL

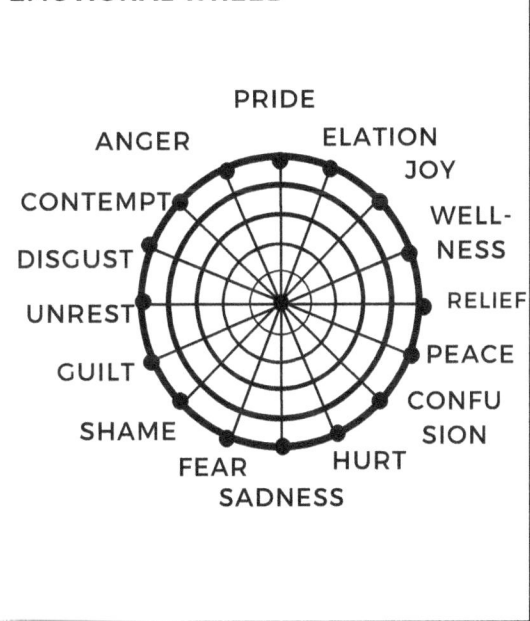

PRIDE

ANGER   ELATION

                              JOY

CONTEMPT

                              WELL-

DISGUST   NESS

UNREST   RELIEF

                              PEACE

GUILT   CONFU

                              SION

SHAME

        FEAR   HURT

        SADNESS

NEXT STEPS

_____

_____

_____

_____

_____

Things to celebrate......

_____

_____

_____

_____

_____

NEXT APPOINTMENT DATE & TIME

Check in

Doctor's APPOINTMENT   DATE _____

HOW AM I FEELING TODAY?

☐ ☐ ☐ ☐ ☐ ☐ ☐ ☐ ☐

NOT GREAT   INCREDIBLE

Doctor's name & info

REASON FOR VISIT

_____

_____

_____

_____

_____

INSTRUCTIONS GUIDE

_____

_____

_____

_____

RESULTS

_____

_____

_____

_____

_____

EMOTIONAL WHEEL

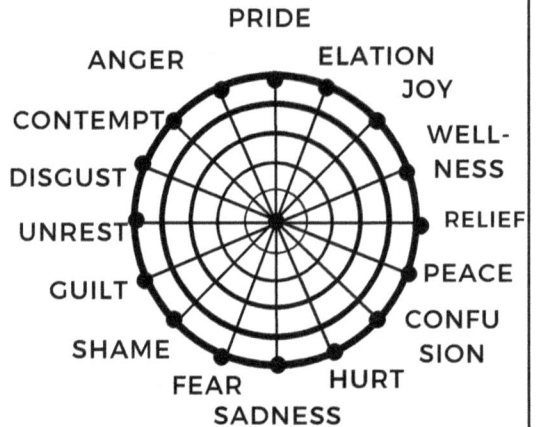

PRIDE
ANGER   ELATION
                  JOY
CONTEMPT
                  WELL-
                  NESS
DISGUST
UNREST   RELIEF
GUILT   PEACE
                  CONFU
SHAME   SION
     FEAR   HURT
     SADNESS

NEXT STEPS

_____

_____

_____

_____

_____

Things to celebrate......

_____

_____

_____

_____

_____

NEXT APPOINTMENT DATE & TIME

Check in

Doctor's APPOINTMENT   DATE _____

HOW AM I FEELING TODAY?

☐ ☐ ☐ ☐ ☐ ☐ ☐ ☐ ☐ ☐

NOT GREAT   INCREDIBLE

Doctor's name &
info

RESULTS

_____
_____
_____
_____
_____

REASON FOR VISIT

_____
_____
_____
_____
_____

INSTRUCTIONS GUIDE

_____
_____
_____

EMOTIONAL WHEEL

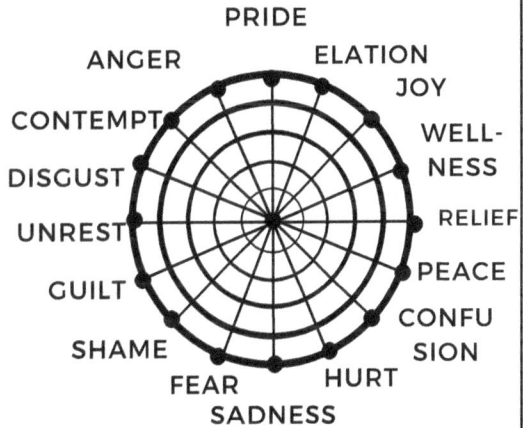

PRIDE
ANGER   ELATION
                JOY
CONTEMPT   WELL-
                      NESS
DISGUST
                    RELIEF
UNREST
                  PEACE
GUILT
              CONFU
SHAME   SION
        FEAR   HURT
      SADNESS

NEXT STEPS

_____
_____
_____
_____

Things to celebrate......

_____
_____
_____
_____

NEXT APPOINTMENT DATE & TIME

Check in

Doctor's APPOINTMENT

DATE _____

HOW AM I FEELING TODAY?

☐ ☐ ☐ ☐ ☐ ☐ ☐ ☐ ☐ ☐

NOT GREAT   INCREDIBLE

Doctor's name & info

REASON FOR VISIT

_____
_____
_____
_____
_____

INSTRUCTIONS GUIDE

_____
_____
_____
_____

RESULTS

_____
_____
_____
_____
_____

EMOTIONAL WHEEL

PRIDE
ANGER   ELATION
                    JOY
CONTEMPT
                WELL-
                NESS
DISGUST
                    RELIEF
UNREST
                PEACE
GUILT
            CONFU
            SION
SHAME
        HURT
    FEAR
    SADNESS

NEXT STEPS

_____
_____
_____
_____
_____

Things to celebrate......

_____
_____
_____
_____

NEXT APPOINTMENT DATE & TIME

Check in

Doctor's APPOINTMENT   DATE _____

HOW AM I FEELING TODAY?

☐ ☐ ☐ ☐ ☐ ☐ ☐ ☐ ☐ ☐

NOT GREAT   INCREDIBLE

Doctor's name &
info

RESULTS

_____
_____
_____
_____
_____
_____

REASON FOR VISIT

_____
_____
_____
_____
_____

EMOTIONAL WHEEL

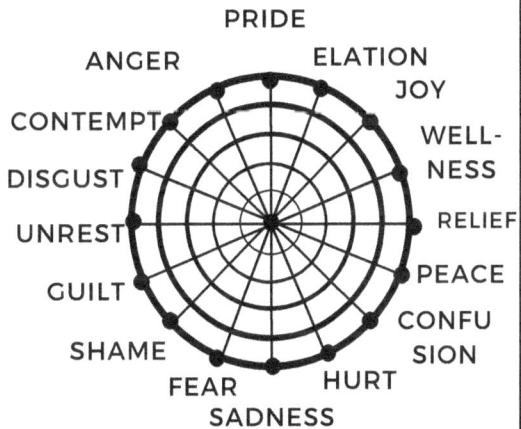

PRIDE

ANGER   ELATION
                    JOY
CONTEMPT
                   WELL-
DISGUST   NESS

UNREST   RELIEF

GUILT   PEACE

SHAME   CONFU
                    SION
          FEAR   HURT
        SADNESS

INSTRUCTIONS GUIDE

_____
_____
_____
_____

NEXT STEPS

_____
_____
_____
_____
_____

Things to celebrate ......

_____
_____
_____
_____
_____

NEXT APPOINTMENT DATE & TIME

Check in

Doctor's APPOINTMENT

DATE _____

HOW AM I FEELING TODAY?

☐ ☐ ☐ ☐ ☐ ☐ ☐ ☐ ☐ ☐

NOT GREAT   INCREDIBLE

Doctor's name & info

REASON FOR VISIT

_____
_____
_____
_____
_____
_____

INSTRUCTIONS GUIDE

_____
_____
_____
_____

RESULTS

_____
_____
_____
_____
_____
_____

EMOTIONAL WHEEL

PRIDE
ANGER   ELATION
                JOY
CONTEMPT
                WELL-
                NESS
DISGUST
                RELIEF
UNREST
                PEACE
GUILT
                CONFU
SHAME   SION
        FEAR   HURT
        SADNESS

NEXT STEPS

_____
_____
_____
_____
_____

Things to celebrate......

_____
_____
_____
_____
_____

NEXT APPOINTMENT DATE & TIME

Check in

Doctor's APPOINTMENT   DATE _____

HOW AM I FEELING TODAY?

☐ ☐ ☐ ☐ ☐ ☐ ☐ ☐ ☐ ☐

NOT GREAT   INCREDIBLE

*Doctor's name &
info*

REASON FOR VISIT

_____

_____

_____

_____

_____

INSTRUCTIONS GUIDE

_____

_____

_____

_____

RESULTS

_____

_____

_____

_____

_____

_____

EMOTIONAL WHEEL

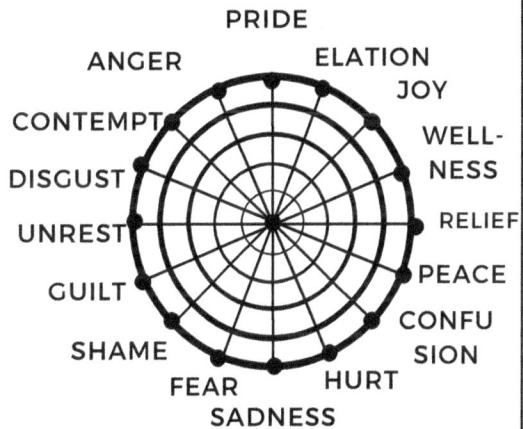

PRIDE

ANGER   ELATION

                    JOY

CONTEMPT

                    WELL-
                    NESS

DISGUST

UNREST   RELIEF

GUILT   PEACE

                    CONFU
SHAME   SION

        FEAR   HURT

        SADNESS

NEXT STEPS

_____

_____

_____

_____

_____

Things to celebrate......

_____

_____

_____

_____

NEXT APPOINTMENT DATE & TIME

Check in

Doctor's APPOINTMENT   DATE _____

HOW AM I FEELING TODAY?

☐ ☐ ☐ ☐ ☐ ☐ ☐ ☐ ☐ ☐

NOT GREAT   INCREDIBLE

Doctor's name & info

REASON FOR VISIT

_____
_____
_____
_____
_____

INSTRUCTIONS GUIDE

_____
_____
_____
_____

RESULTS

_____
_____
_____
_____
_____

EMOTIONAL WHEEL

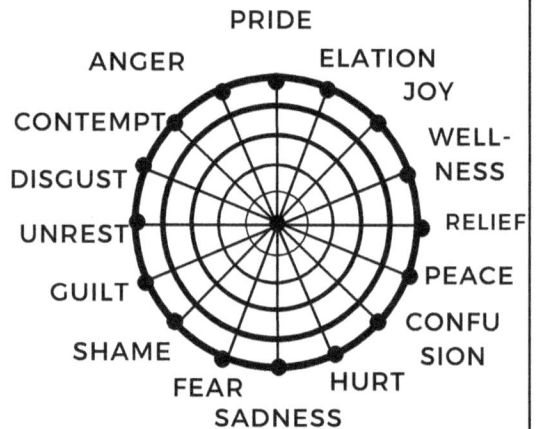

PRIDE
ANGER   ELATION
                        JOY
CONTEMPT
                     WELL-
                     NESS
DISGUST
                        RELIEF
UNREST
                     PEACE
GUILT
                    CONFU
SHAME   SION
        FEAR   HURT
        SADNESS

NEXT STEPS

_____
_____
_____
_____
_____

Things to celebrate......

_____
_____
_____
_____

NEXT APPOINTMENT DATE & TIME

Check in

Doctor's APPOINTMENT   DATE _____

HOW AM I FEELING TODAY?

☐ ☐ ☐ ☐ ☐ ☐ ☐ ☐ ☐ ☐

NOT GREAT   INCREDIBLE

Doctor's name & info

REASON FOR VISIT

_____

_____

_____

_____

_____

INSTRUCTIONS GUIDE

_____

_____

_____

_____

RESULTS

_____

_____

_____

_____

_____

EMOTIONAL WHEEL

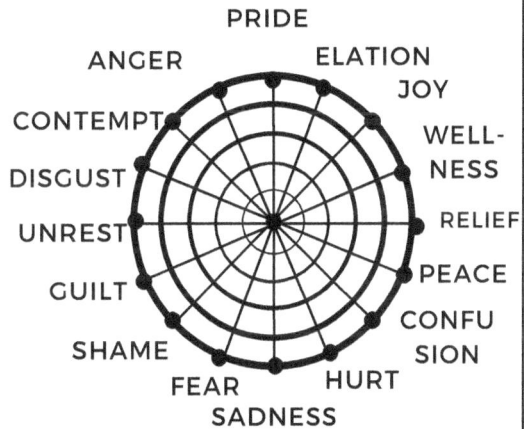

PRIDE

ANGER   ELATION

                    JOY

CONTEMPT

                    WELL-
                    NESS
DISGUST

UNREST   RELIEF

                    PEACE
GUILT
                    CONFU
SHAME   SION

        FEAR   HURT
        SADNESS

NEXT STEPS

_____

_____

_____

_____

_____

Things to celebrate......

_____

_____

_____

_____

NEXT APPOINTMENT DATE & TIME

Check in

Doctor's APPOINTMENT

DATE _____

HOW AM I FEELING TODAY?

☐ ☐ ☐ ☐ ☐ ☐ ☐ ☐ ☐ ☐

NOT GREAT   INCREDIBLE

Doctor's name & info

REASON FOR VISIT

_____
_____
_____
_____
_____

INSTRUCTIONS GUIDE

_____
_____
_____
_____

RESULTS

_____
_____
_____
_____
_____

EMOTIONAL WHEEL

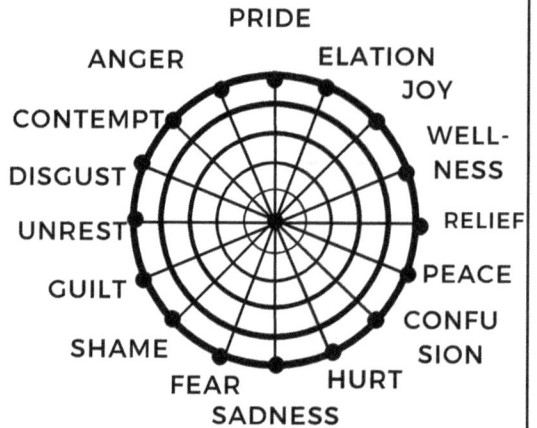

PRIDE
ANGER   ELATION
                JOY
CONTEMPT
                WELL-
                NESS
DISGUST
                RELIEF
UNREST
                PEACE
GUILT
                CONFU
SHAME   SION
        FEAR   HURT
        SADNESS

NEXT STEPS

_____
_____
_____
_____
_____

Things to celebrate......

_____
_____
_____
_____
_____

NEXT APPOINTMENT DATE & TIME

Check in

Doctor's APPOINTMENT   DATE _____

HOW AM I FEELING TODAY?

☐ ☐ ☐ ☐ ☐ ☐ ☐ ☐ ☐ ☐

NOT GREAT   INCREDIBLE

Doctor's name &
info

REASON FOR VISIT

_____

_____

_____

_____

_____

_____

INSTRUCTIONS GUIDE

_____

_____

_____

_____

NEXT STEPS

_____

_____

_____

_____

_____

RESULTS

_____

_____

_____

_____

_____

EMOTIONAL WHEEL

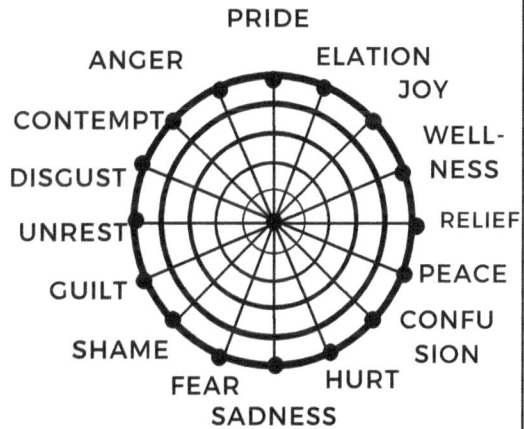

PRIDE

ANGER   ELATION
                JOY

CONTEMPT   WELL-
                      NESS

DISGUST

UNREST   RELIEF

GUILT   PEACE

SHAME   CONFU
                    SION

FEAR   HURT
SADNESS

Things to celebrate ......

_____

_____

_____

_____

_____

NEXT APPOINTMENT DATE & TIME

Check in

Doctor's APPOINTMENT   DATE _____

HOW AM I FEELING TODAY?

☐ ☐ ☐ ☐ ☐ ☐ ☐ ☐ ☐ ☐

NOT GREAT   INCREDIBLE

Doctor's name &
info

REASON FOR VISIT

_____
_____
_____
_____
_____

INSTRUCTIONS GUIDE

_____
_____
_____
_____

NEXT STEPS

_____
_____
_____
_____
_____

RESULTS

_____
_____
_____
_____
_____

EMOTIONAL WHEEL

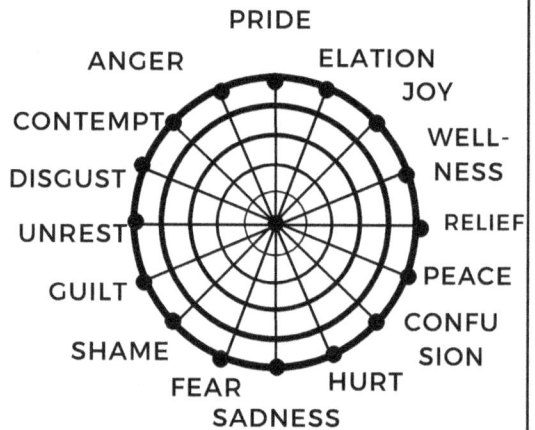

PRIDE

ANGER   ELATION

                              JOY

CONTEMPT

                         WELL-
                         NESS

DISGUST

                              RELIEF

UNREST

                              PEACE

GUILT

                         CONFU
                         SION

SHAME

FEAR   HURT

SADNESS

Things to celebrate......

_____
_____
_____
_____

NEXT APPOINTMENT DATE & TIME

Check in

Doctor's APPOINTMENT   DATE _____

HOW AM I FEELING TODAY?

☐ ☐ ☐ ☐ ☐ ☐ ☐ ☐ ☐ ☐

NOT GREAT   INCREDIBLE

Doctor's name & info

REASON FOR VISIT

_____

_____

_____

_____

_____

INSTRUCTIONS GUIDE

_____

_____

_____

_____

NEXT STEPS

_____

_____

_____

_____

_____

RESULTS

_____

_____

_____

_____

_____

EMOTIONAL WHEEL

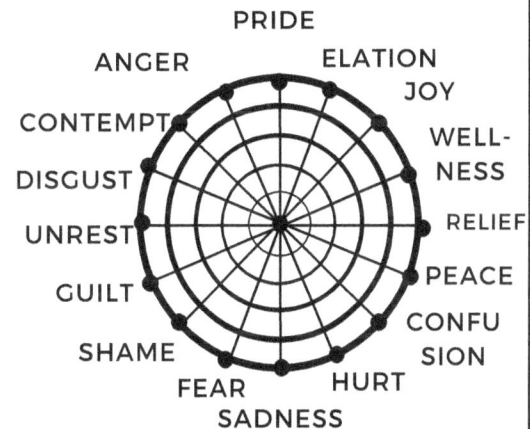

PRIDE

ANGER   ELATION

JOY

CONTEMPT

WELL-NESS

DISGUST

UNREST   RELIEF

GUILT   PEACE

SHAME   CONFU-SION

FEAR   HURT

SADNESS

Things to celebrate ......

_____

_____

_____

_____

NEXT APPOINTMENT DATE & TIME

Check in

Doctor's APPOINTMENT DATE _____

HOW AM I FEELING TODAY?

☐ ☐ ☐ ☐ ☐ ☐ ☐ ☐ ☐ ☐

NOT GREAT   INCREDIBLE

Doctor's name & info

REASON FOR VISIT

_____
_____
_____
_____
_____

INSTRUCTIONS GUIDE

_____
_____
_____
_____

NEXT STEPS

_____
_____
_____
_____
_____

RESULTS

_____
_____
_____
_____
_____

EMOTIONAL WHEEL

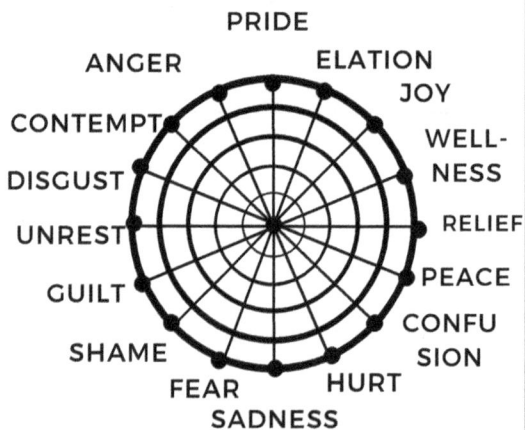

PRIDE
ANGER   ELATION
                      JOY
CONTEMPT
                   WELL-
DISGUST   NESS
UNREST   RELIEF
                   PEACE
GUILT   CONFU
SHAME   SION
    FEAR   HURT
    SADNESS

Things to celebrate ......

_____
_____
_____
_____
_____

NEXT APPOINTMENT DATE & TIME

Check in

Doctor's APPOINTMENT   DATE _____

HOW AM I FEELING TODAY?

☐ ☐ ☐ ☐ ☐ ☐ ☐ ☐ ☐ ☐

NOT GREAT   INCREDIBLE

Doctor's name & info

REASON FOR VISIT

_____
_____
_____
_____
_____
_____

INSTRUCTIONS GUIDE

_____
_____
_____
_____

RESULTS

_____
_____
_____
_____
_____

EMOTIONAL WHEEL

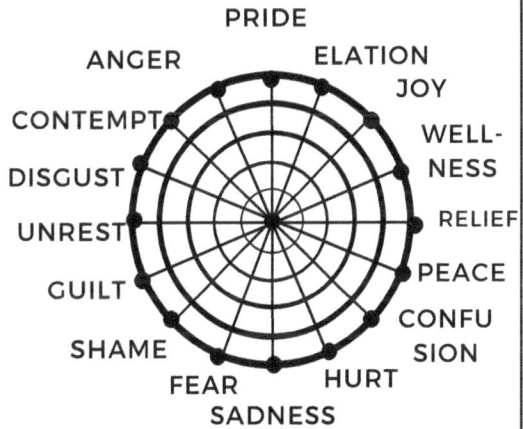

PRIDE
ANGER   ELATION
               JOY
CONTEMPT   WELL-
               NESS
DISGUST
UNREST   RELIEF
GUILT   PEACE
               CONFU
SHAME   SION
FEAR   HURT
SADNESS

NEXT STEPS

_____
_____
_____
_____
_____

Things to celebrate......

_____
_____
_____
_____
_____

NEXT APPOINTMENT DATE & TIME

Check in

Doctor's APPOINTMENT   DATE _____

HOW AM I FEELING TODAY?

☐ ☐ ☐ ☐ ☐ ☐ ☐ ☐ ☐ ☐

NOT GREAT   INCREDIBLE

Doctor's name & info

REASON FOR VISIT

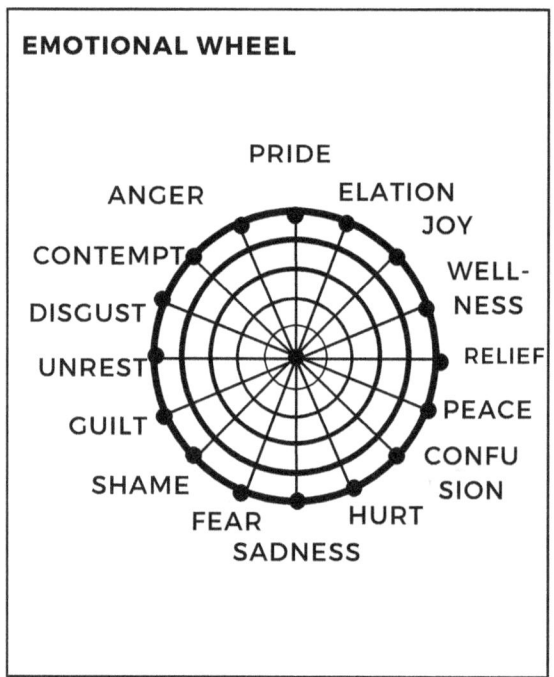

_____
_____
_____
_____
_____

INSTRUCTIONS GUIDE

_____
_____
_____
_____

RESULTS

_____
_____
_____
_____
_____

EMOTIONAL WHEEL

PRIDE
ANGER   ELATION
                        JOY
CONTEMPT
                     WELL-
                     NESS
DISGUST
UNREST   RELIEF
                        PEACE
GUILT   CONFU
                     SION
SHAME
        FEAR   HURT
        SADNESS

NEXT STEPS

_____
_____
_____
_____
_____

Things to celebrate......

_____
_____
_____
_____

NEXT APPOINTMENT DATE & TIME

Check in

Doctor's APPOINTMENT   DATE _____

HOW AM I FEELING TODAY?

☐ ☐ ☐ ☐ ☐ ☐ ☐ ☐ ☐ ☐

NOT GREAT   INCREDIBLE

Doctor's name & info

REASON FOR VISIT

_____
_____
_____
_____
_____

INSTRUCTIONS GUIDE

_____
_____
_____
_____

RESULTS

_____
_____
_____
_____
_____
_____

EMOTIONAL WHEEL

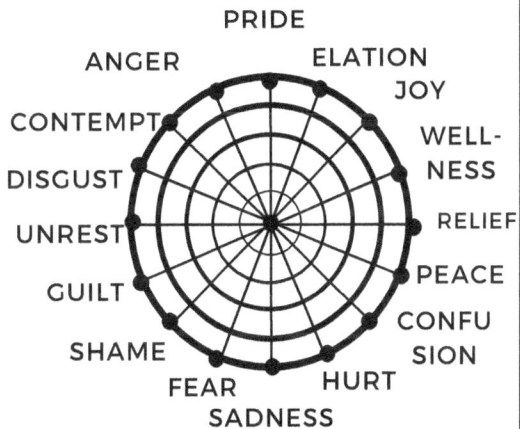

PRIDE
ANGER   ELATION
                JOY
CONTEMPT
                WELL-
                NESS
DISGUST
                RELIEF
UNREST
                PEACE
GUILT
                CONFU
SHAME   SION
      FEAR   HURT
      SADNESS

NEXT STEPS

_____
_____
_____
_____
_____

Things to celebrate......

_____
_____
_____
_____
_____

NEXT APPOINTMENT DATE & TIME

Check in

Doctor's APPOINTMENT DATE _____

HOW AM I FEELING TODAY?

☐ ☐ ☐ ☐ ☐ ☐ ☐ ☐ ☐ ☐

NOT GREAT   INCREDIBLE

Doctor's name & info

REASON FOR VISIT

_____
_____
_____
_____
_____
_____

INSTRUCTIONS GUIDE

_____
_____
_____
_____

RESULTS

_____
_____
_____
_____
_____

EMOTIONAL WHEEL

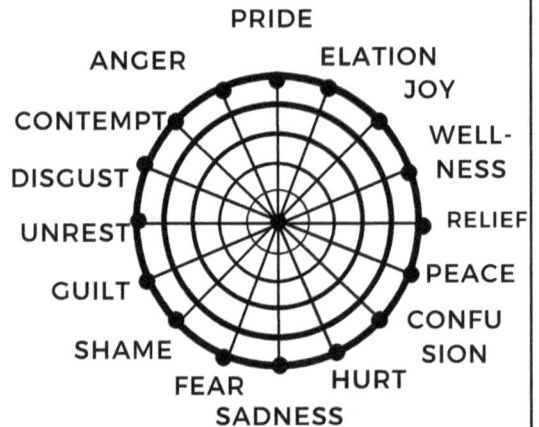

PRIDE
ANGER   ELATION
                JOY
CONTEMPT
                WELL-
DISGUST   NESS

UNREST   RELIEF

GUILT   PEACE
                CONFU
SHAME   SION
       FEAR HURT
        SADNESS

NEXT STEPS

_____
_____
_____
_____
_____

Things to celebrate......

_____
_____
_____
_____
_____

NEXT APPOINTMENT DATE & TIME

Check in

Doctor's APPOINTMENT   DATE _____

HOW AM I FEELING TODAY?

☐ ☐ ☐ ☐ ☐ ☐ ☐ ☐ ☐ ☐

NOT GREAT   INCREDIBLE

Doctor's name & info

REASON FOR VISIT

_____
_____
_____
_____
_____

INSTRUCTIONS GUIDE

_____
_____
_____
_____

RESULTS

_____
_____
_____
_____
_____
_____

EMOTIONAL WHEEL

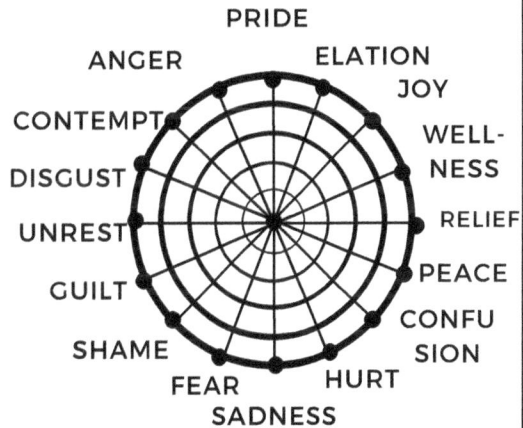

PRIDE
ANGER   ELATION
                        JOY
CONTEMPT   WELL-
                            NESS
DISGUST
                       RELIEF
UNREST
                    PEACE
GUILT   CONFU
                    SION
SHAME
    FEAR   HURT
    SADNESS

NEXT STEPS

_____
_____
_____
_____
_____

Things to celebrate......

_____
_____
_____
_____
_____

NEXT APPOINTMENT DATE & TIME

Check in

Doctor's APPOINTMENT   DATE _____

HOW AM I FEELING TODAY?

☐ ☐ ☐ ☐ ☐ ☐ ☐ ☐ ☐ ☐

NOT GREAT   INCREDIBLE

Doctor's name &
info

RESULTS

_____
_____
_____
_____
_____
_____

REASON FOR VISIT

_____
_____
_____
_____
_____

EMOTIONAL WHEEL

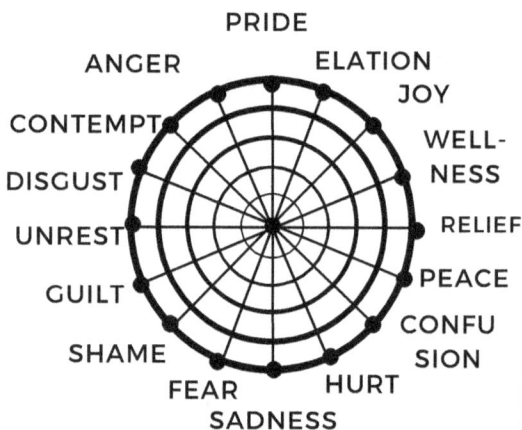

PRIDE

ANGER   ELATION
                              JOY
CONTEMPT
                              WELL-
DISGUST   NESS

UNREST   RELIEF

GUILT   PEACE

                              CONFU
SHAME   SION

        FEAR   HURT
        SADNESS

INSTRUCTIONS GUIDE

_____
_____
_____
_____

NEXT STEPS

_____
_____
_____
_____
_____

Things to celebrate ......

_____
_____
_____
_____

NEXT APPOINTMENT DATE & TIME

Check in

Doctor's APPOINTMENT   DATE _____

HOW AM I FEELING TODAY?

☐ ☐ ☐ ☐ ☐ ☐ ☐ ☐ ☐ ☐

NOT GREAT   INCREDIBLE

Doctor's name & info

REASON FOR VISIT

_____

_____

_____

_____

_____

INSTRUCTIONS GUIDE

_____

_____

_____

_____

NEXT STEPS

_____

_____

_____

_____

RESULTS

_____

_____

_____

_____

_____

EMOTIONAL WHEEL

PRIDE

ANGER   ELATION

JOY

CONTEMPT   WELL-
NESS

DISGUST

RELIEF

UNREST

PEACE

GUILT   CONFU
SION

SHAME

FEAR   HURT

SADNESS

Things to celebrate ......

_____

_____

_____

_____

_____

NEXT APPOINTMENT DATE & TIME

Check in

Doctor's APPOINTMENT

DATE _____

HOW AM I FEELING TODAY?

☐ ☐ ☐ ☐ ☐ ☐ ☐ ☐ ☐

NOT GREAT   INCREDIBLE

Doctor's name & info

REASON FOR VISIT

_____

_____

_____

_____

_____

INSTRUCTIONS GUIDE

_____

_____

_____

_____

RESULTS

_____

_____

_____

_____

_____

EMOTIONAL WHEEL

PRIDE
ANGER
ELATION
JOY
CONTEMPT
WELL-NESS
DISGUST
UNREST
RELIEF
GUILT
PEACE
SHAME
CONFUSION
FEAR
HURT
SADNESS

NEXT STEPS

_____

_____

_____

_____

Things to celebrate......

_____

_____

_____

_____

_____

NEXT APPOINTMENT DATE & TIME

Check in

Doctor's APPOINTMENT   DATE _____

HOW AM I FEELING TODAY?

☐ ☐ ☐ ☐ ☐ ☐ ☐ ☐ ☐ ☐

NOT GREAT   INCREDIBLE

Doctor's name & info

REASON FOR VISIT

_____

_____

_____

_____

_____

INSTRUCTIONS GUIDE

_____

_____

_____

_____

RESULTS

_____

_____

_____

_____

_____

EMOTIONAL WHEEL

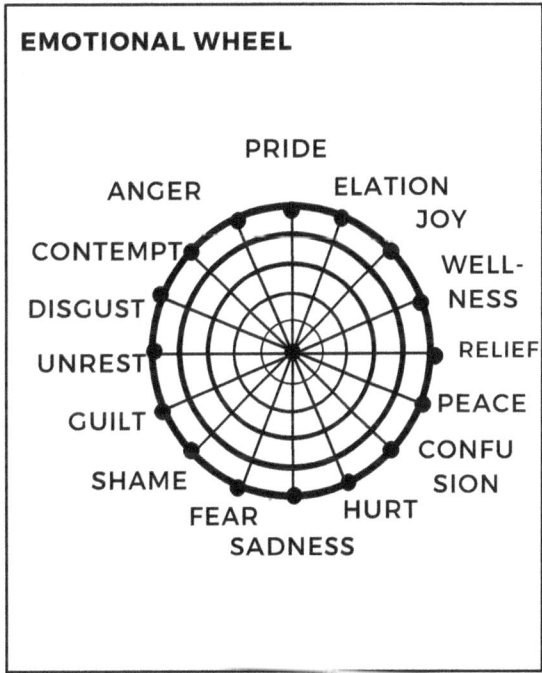

PRIDE

ANGER   ELATION

JOY

CONTEMPT   WELL-NESS

DISGUST

UNREST   RELIEF

GUILT   PEACE

CONFU SION

SHAME   HURT

FEAR

SADNESS

NEXT STEPS

_____

_____

_____

_____

_____

Things to celebrate......

_____

_____

_____

_____

NEXT APPOINTMENT DATE & TIME

Check in

Doctor's APPOINTMENT   DATE _____

HOW AM I FEELING TODAY?

☐ ☐ ☐ ☐ ☐ ☐ ☐ ☐ ☐ ☐

NOT GREAT   INCREDIBLE

Doctor's name & info

REASON FOR VISIT

_____
_____
_____
_____
_____

INSTRUCTIONS GUIDE

_____
_____
_____
_____

RESULTS

_____
_____
_____
_____
_____

EMOTIONAL WHEEL

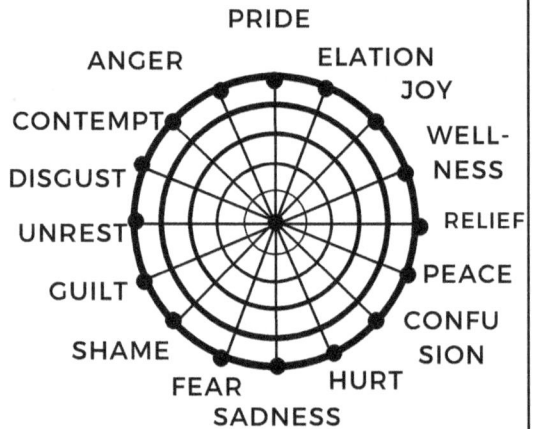

PRIDE
ANGER   ELATION
                JOY
CONTEMPT
                WELL-
DISGUST   NESS
UNREST   RELIEF
GUILT   PEACE
                CONFU
SHAME   SION
        FEAR   HURT
        SADNESS

NEXT STEPS

_____
_____
_____
_____
_____

Things to celebrate......

_____
_____
_____
_____

NEXT APPOINTMENT DATE & TIME

Check in

Doctor's APPOINTMENT   DATE _____

HOW AM I FEELING TODAY?

☐ ☐ ☐ ☐ ☐ ☐ ☐ ☐ ☐ ☐

NOT GREAT   INCREDIBLE

Doctor's name & info

REASON FOR VISIT

_____
_____
_____
_____
_____

INSTRUCTIONS GUIDE

_____
_____
_____
_____

NEXT STEPS

_____
_____
_____
_____
_____

RESULTS

_____
_____
_____
_____
_____
_____

EMOTIONAL WHEEL

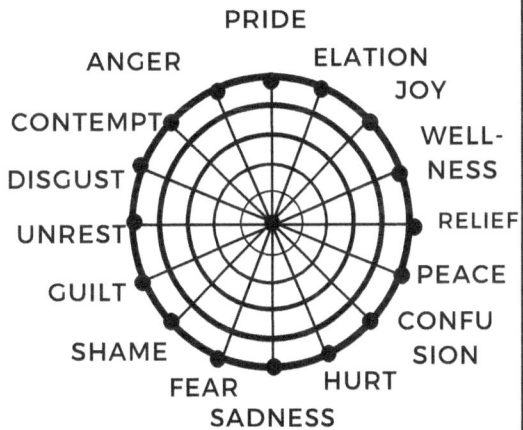

PRIDE
ANGER   ELATION
                    JOY
CONTEMPT   WELL-
                    NESS
DISGUST
                 RELIEF
UNREST
                 PEACE
GUILT   CONFU
                    SION
SHAME
      FEAR   HURT
      SADNESS

Things to celebrate ......

_____
_____
_____
_____
_____

NEXT APPOINTMENT DATE & TIME

Check in

Doctor's APPOINTMENT   DATE _____

HOW AM I FEELING TODAY?

☐ ☐ ☐ ☐ ☐ ☐ ☐ ☐ ☐ ☐

NOT GREAT   INCREDIBLE

Doctor's name &
info

REASON FOR VISIT

_____
_____
_____
_____
_____

INSTRUCTIONS GUIDE

_____
_____
_____
_____

RESULTS

_____
_____
_____
_____
_____

EMOTIONAL WHEEL

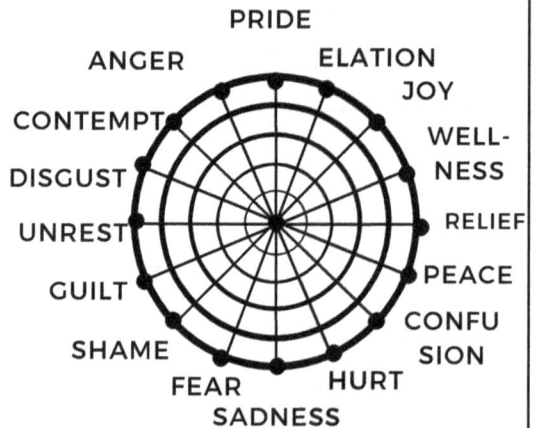

PRIDE
ANGER   ELATION
                              JOY
CONTEMPT
                         WELL-
DISGUST   NESS
UNREST   RELIEF
GUILT   PEACE
                         CONFU
SHAME   SION
       FEAR   HURT
         SADNESS

NEXT STEPS

_____
_____
_____
_____
_____

Things to celebrate......

_____
_____
_____
_____

NEXT APPOINTMENT DATE & TIME

Check in

Doctor's APPOINTMENT   DATE _____

HOW AM I FEELING TODAY?

☐ ☐ ☐ ☐ ☐ ☐ ☐ ☐ ☐ ☐

NOT GREAT   INCREDIBLE

Doctor's name &
info

REASON FOR VISIT

_____

_____

_____

_____

_____

_____

INSTRUCTIONS GUIDE

_____

_____

_____

_____

NEXT STEPS

_____

_____

_____

_____

_____

RESULTS

_____

_____

_____

_____

_____

EMOTIONAL WHEEL

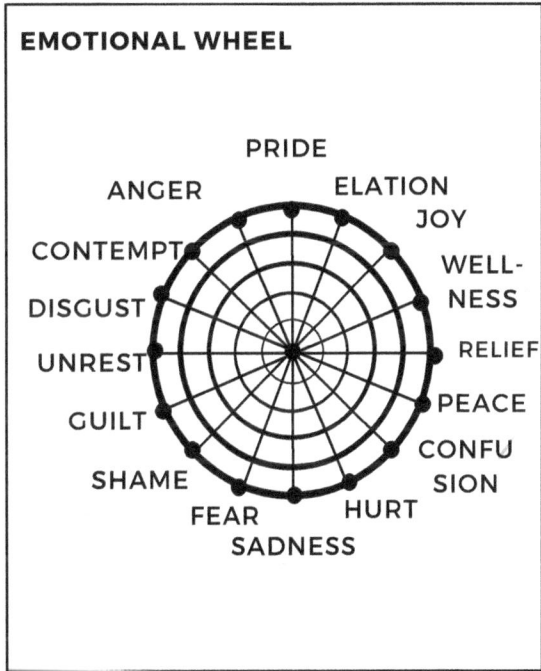

PRIDE
ANGER   ELATION
                    JOY
CONTEMPT   WELL-
                          NESS
DISGUST
                       RELIEF
UNREST
                      PEACE
GUILT
                    CONFU
SHAME   SION
        FEAR   HURT
        SADNESS

Things to celebrate ......

_____

_____

_____

_____

_____

NEXT APPOINTMENT DATE & TIME

Check in

Doctor's APPOINTMENT   DATE _____

HOW AM I FEELING TODAY?

☐ ☐ ☐ ☐ ☐ ☐ ☐ ☐ ☐ ☐

NOT GREAT   INCREDIBLE

Doctor's name & info

REASON FOR VISIT

_____

_____

_____

_____

_____

INSTRUCTIONS GUIDE

_____

_____

_____

_____

NEXT STEPS

_____

_____

_____

_____

_____

RESULTS

_____

_____

_____

_____

_____

_____

EMOTIONAL WHEEL

PRIDE

ANGER   ELATION

JOY

CONTEMPT

WELL-NESS

DISGUST

UNREST   RELIEF

PEACE

GUILT   CONFU

SION

SHAME   HURT

FEAR

SADNESS

Things to celebrate......

_____

_____

_____

_____

_____

NEXT APPOINTMENT DATE & TIME

Check in

Doctor's APPOINTMENT   DATE _____

HOW AM I FEELING TODAY?

☐ ☐ ☐ ☐ ☐ ☐ ☐ ☐ ☐ ☐

NOT GREAT   INCREDIBLE

Doctor's name & info

REASON FOR VISIT

_____
_____
_____
_____
_____

INSTRUCTIONS GUIDE

_____
_____
_____
_____

NEXT STEPS

_____
_____
_____
_____
_____

RESULTS

_____
_____
_____
_____
_____
_____

EMOTIONAL WHEEL

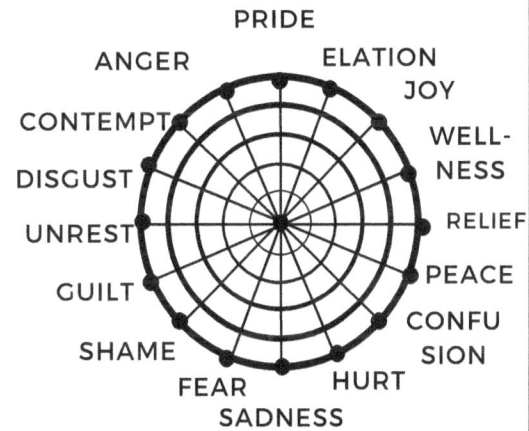

PRIDE
ANGER   ELATION
     JOY
CONTEMPT
    WELL-
    NESS
DISGUST
    RELIEF
UNREST
    PEACE
GUILT
   CONFU
   SION
SHAME
    HURT
FEAR
SADNESS

Things to celebrate......

_____
_____
_____
_____
_____

NEXT APPOINTMENT DATE & TIME

Check in

Doctor's APPOINTMENT   DATE _____

HOW AM I FEELING TODAY?

☐ ☐ ☐ ☐ ☐ ☐ ☐ ☐ ☐ ☐

NOT GREAT   INCREDIBLE

Doctor's name & info

REASON FOR VISIT

_____
_____
_____
_____
_____

INSTRUCTIONS GUIDE

_____
_____
_____
_____

RESULTS

_____
_____
_____
_____
_____

EMOTIONAL WHEEL

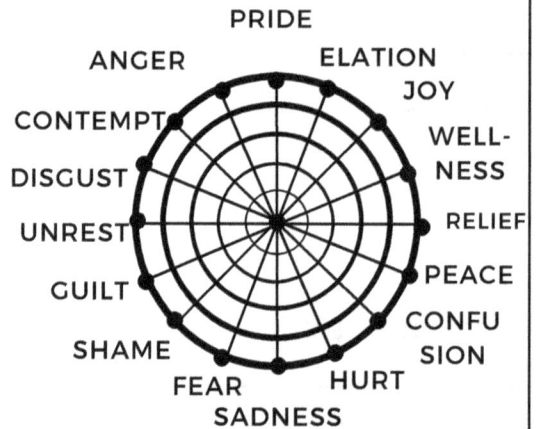

PRIDE

ANGER   ELATION
                        JOY
CONTEMPT
                    WELL-
DISGUST   NESS

UNREST   RELIEF

GUILT   PEACE

SHAME   CONFU
                   SION
      FEAR   HURT
      SADNESS

NEXT STEPS

_____
_____
_____
_____
_____

Things to celebrate ......

_____
_____
_____
_____
_____

NEXT APPOINTMENT DATE & TIME

Check in

Doctor's APPOINTMENT   DATE _____

HOW AM I FEELING TODAY?

☐ ☐ ☐ ☐ ☐ ☐ ☐ ☐ ☐ ☐

NOT GREAT   INCREDIBLE

Doctor's name & info

REASON FOR VISIT

_____

_____

_____

_____

_____

INSTRUCTIONS GUIDE

_____

_____

_____

_____

NEXT STEPS

_____

_____

_____

_____

_____

RESULTS

_____

_____

_____

_____

_____

EMOTIONAL WHEEL

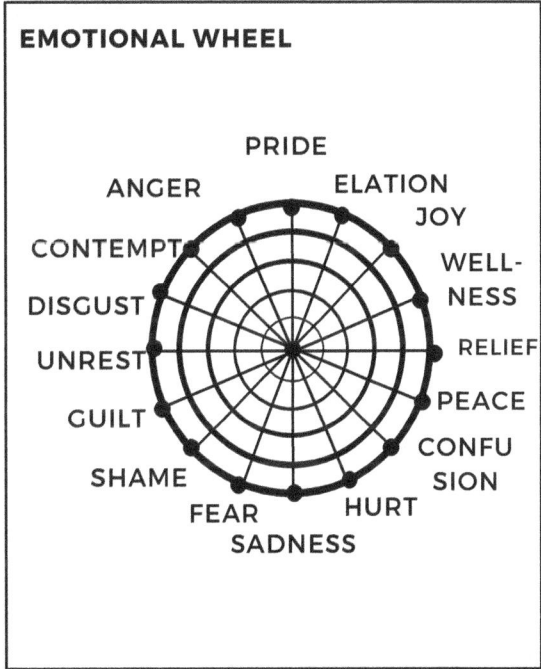

PRIDE
ANGER   ELATION
JOY
CONTEMPT   WELL-NESS
DISGUST
RELIEF
UNREST
PEACE
GUILT   CONFU
SION
SHAME
HURT
FEAR
SADNESS

Things to celebrate......

_____

_____

_____

_____

NEXT APPOINTMENT DATE & TIME

Check in

Doctor's APPOINTMENT   DATE _____

HOW AM I FEELING TODAY?

☐ ☐ ☐ ☐ ☐ ☐ ☐ ☐ ☐

NOT GREAT   INCREDIBLE

Doctor's name & info

REASON FOR VISIT

_____
_____
_____
_____
_____

INSTRUCTIONS GUIDE

_____
_____
_____
_____

NEXT STEPS

_____
_____
_____
_____
_____

RESULTS

_____
_____
_____
_____
_____

EMOTIONAL WHEEL

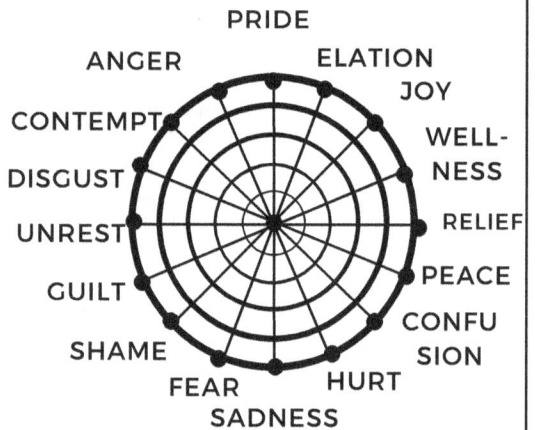

PRIDE
ANGER   ELATION
                JOY
CONTEMPT
                WELL-
DISGUST   NESS

UNREST   RELIEF

GUILT   PEACE
              CONFU
SHAME   SION
      FEAR   HURT
      SADNESS

Things to celebrate......

_____
_____
_____
_____
_____

NEXT APPOINTMENT DATE & TIME

Check in

Doctor's APPOINTMENT   DATE _____

HOW AM I FEELING TODAY?

☐ ☐ ☐ ☐ ☐ ☐ ☐ ☐ ☐ ☐

NOT GREAT   INCREDIBLE

Doctor's name &
info

RESULTS

_____
_____
_____
_____
_____
_____

REASON FOR VISIT

_____
_____
_____
_____
_____

EMOTIONAL WHEEL

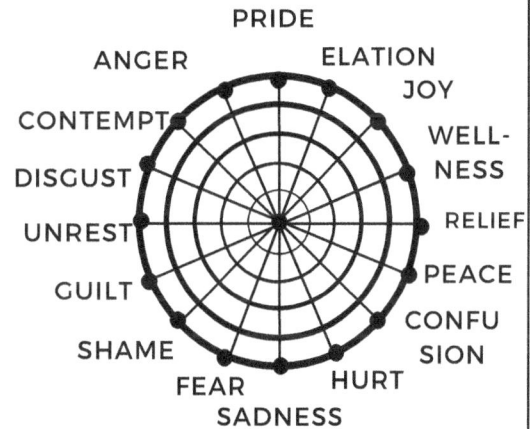

PRIDE
ANGER   ELATION
                    JOY
CONTEMPT
                 WELL-
DISGUST   NESS
UNREST   RELIEF
GUILT   PEACE
                 CONFU
SHAME   SION
     FEAR   HURT
      SADNESS

INSTRUCTIONS GUIDE

_____
_____
_____
_____

NEXT STEPS

_____
_____
_____
_____
_____

Things to celebrate......

_____
_____
_____
_____

NEXT APPOINTMENT DATE & TIME

Check in

Doctor's APPOINTMENT   DATE _____

HOW AM I FEELING TODAY?

☐ ☐ ☐ ☐ ☐ ☐ ☐ ☐ ☐ ☐

NOT GREAT   INCREDIBLE

Doctor's name & info

REASON FOR VISIT

_____
_____
_____
_____
_____

INSTRUCTIONS GUIDE

_____
_____
_____
_____

RESULTS

_____
_____
_____
_____
_____

EMOTIONAL WHEEL

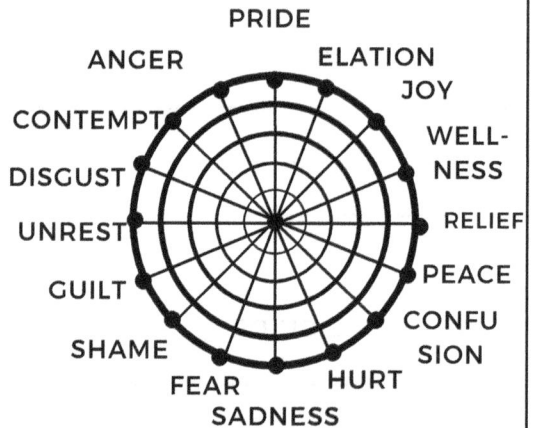

PRIDE

ANGER   ELATION
                              JOY

CONTEMPT

DISGUST   WELL-
                           NESS

UNREST   RELIEF

GUILT   PEACE

                          CONFU
SHAME   SION

        FEAR   HURT
        SADNESS

NEXT STEPS

_____
_____
_____
_____
_____

Things to celebrate .....

_____
_____
_____
_____

NEXT APPOINTMENT DATE & TIME

Check in

Doctor's APPOINTMENT   DATE _____

HOW AM I FEELING TODAY?

☐ ☐ ☐ ☐ ☐ ☐ ☐ ☐ ☐ ☐

NOT GREAT   INCREDIBLE

Doctor's name & info

REASON FOR VISIT

_____
_____
_____
_____
_____

INSTRUCTIONS GUIDE

_____
_____
_____
_____

NEXT STEPS

_____
_____
_____
_____

RESULTS

_____
_____
_____
_____
_____

EMOTIONAL WHEEL

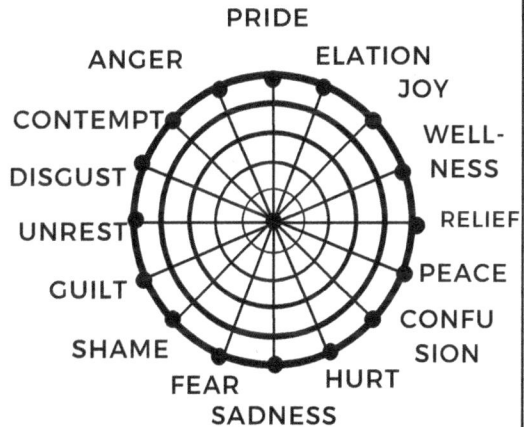

PRIDE
ANGER   ELATION
JOY
CONTEMPT   WELL-NESS
DISGUST
UNREST   RELIEF
GUILT   PEACE
SHAME   CONFU SION
FEAR   HURT
SADNESS

Things to celebrate......

_____
_____
_____
_____

NEXT APPOINTMENT DATE & TIME

Check in

Doctor's APPOINTMENT   DATE _____

HOW AM I FEELING TODAY?

☐ ☐ ☐ ☐ ☐ ☐ ☐ ☐ ☐

NOT GREAT   INCREDIBLE

Doctor's name & info

REASON FOR VISIT

_____
_____
_____
_____
_____
_____

INSTRUCTIONS GUIDE

_____
_____
_____
_____

RESULTS

_____
_____
_____
_____
_____

EMOTIONAL WHEEL

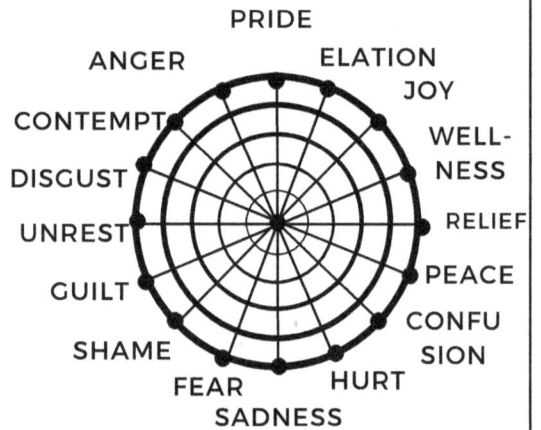

PRIDE
ANGER   ELATION
                    JOY
CONTEMPT
                WELL-
DISGUST   NESS
UNREST   RELIEF
GUILT   PEACE
                CONFU
SHAME   SION
    FEAR   HURT
    SADNESS

NEXT STEPS

_____
_____
_____
_____
_____

Things to celebrate......

_____
_____
_____
_____
_____

NEXT APPOINTMENT DATE & TIME

Check in

Doctor's APPOINTMENT   DATE _____

HOW AM I FEELING TODAY?

☐ ☐ ☐ ☐ ☐ ☐ ☐ ☐ ☐ ☐

NOT GREAT   INCREDIBLE

Doctor's name &
info

REASON FOR VISIT

_____

_____

_____

_____

_____

INSTRUCTIONS GUIDE

_____

_____

_____

_____

NEXT STEPS

_____

_____

_____

_____

_____

RESULTS

_____

_____

_____

_____

_____

_____

EMOTIONAL WHEEL

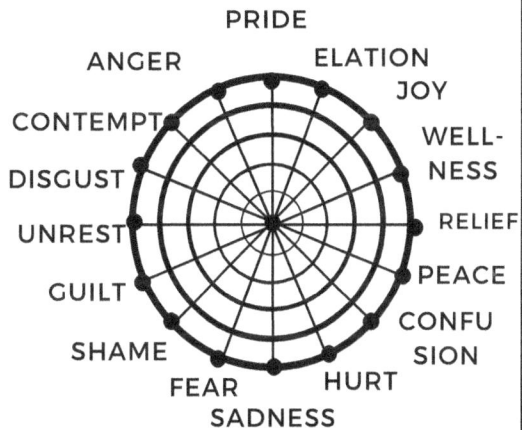

PRIDE
ANGER   ELATION
                        JOY
CONTEMPT
                    WELL-
                    NESS
DISGUST
                    RELIEF
UNREST
                    PEACE
GUILT
                CONFU
SHAME   SION
        FEAR   HURT
        SADNESS

Things to celebrate......

_____

_____

_____

_____

_____

NEXT APPOINTMENT DATE & TIME

Check in

Doctor's APPOINTMENT   DATE _____

HOW AM I FEELING TODAY?

☐ ☐ ☐ ☐ ☐ ☐ ☐ ☐ ☐ ☐

NOT GREAT   INCREDIBLE

Doctor's name & info

REASON FOR VISIT

_____

_____

_____

_____

_____

INSTRUCTIONS GUIDE

_____

_____

_____

_____

RESULTS

_____

_____

_____

_____

_____

EMOTIONAL WHEEL

PRIDE
ANGER   ELATION
                  JOY
CONTEMPT
                  WELL-
DISGUST   NESS
                  RELIEF
UNREST
                  PEACE
GUILT
                  CONFU
SHAME   SION
        FEAR   HURT
        SADNESS

NEXT STEPS

_____

_____

_____

_____

_____

Things to celebrate ......

_____

_____

_____

_____

_____

NEXT APPOINTMENT DATE & TIME

Check in

Doctor's APPOINTMENT   DATE _____

HOW AM I FEELING TODAY?

☐ ☐ ☐ ☐ ☐ ☐ ☐ ☐ ☐

NOT GREAT   INCREDIBLE

Doctor's name & info

REASON FOR VISIT

_____
_____
_____
_____
_____
_____

INSTRUCTIONS GUIDE

_____
_____
_____
_____

NEXT STEPS

_____
_____
_____
_____
_____

RESULTS

_____
_____
_____
_____
_____
_____

EMOTIONAL WHEEL

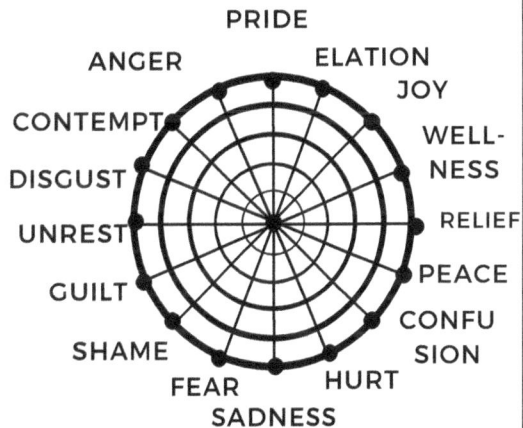

PRIDE

ANGER   ELATION

                JOY

CONTEMPT   WELL-
                    NESS

DISGUST

                    RELIEF

UNREST

                    PEACE

GUILT

                CONFU
                SION

SHAME

        FEAR   HURT

    SADNESS

Things to celebrate......

_____
_____
_____
_____
_____

NEXT APPOINTMENT DATE & TIME

Check in

Doctor's APPOINTMENT   DATE _____

HOW AM I FEELING TODAY?

☐ ☐ ☐ ☐ ☐ ☐ ☐ ☐ ☐ ☐

NOT GREAT   INCREDIBLE

*Doctor's name &
info*

REASON FOR VISIT

_____
_____
_____
_____
_____

INSTRUCTIONS GUIDE

_____
_____
_____
_____

RESULTS

_____
_____
_____
_____
_____

EMOTIONAL WHEEL

PRIDE
ANGER   ELATION
                JOY
CONTEMPT   WELL-
                NESS
DISGUST
UNREST   RELIEF
GUILT   PEACE
                CONFU
SHAME   SION
      FEAR   HURT
      SADNESS

NEXT STEPS

_____
_____
_____
_____
_____

Things to celebrate ......

_____
_____
_____
_____

NEXT APPOINTMENT DATE & TIME

Check in

Doctor's APPOINTMENT   DATE _____

HOW AM I FEELING TODAY?

☐ ☐ ☐ ☐ ☐ ☐ ☐ ☐ ☐

NOT GREAT   INCREDIBLE

Doctor's name & info

REASON FOR VISIT

_____
_____
_____
_____
_____

INSTRUCTIONS GUIDE

_____
_____
_____
_____

NEXT STEPS

_____
_____
_____
_____
_____

RESULTS

_____
_____
_____
_____
_____
_____

EMOTIONAL WHEEL

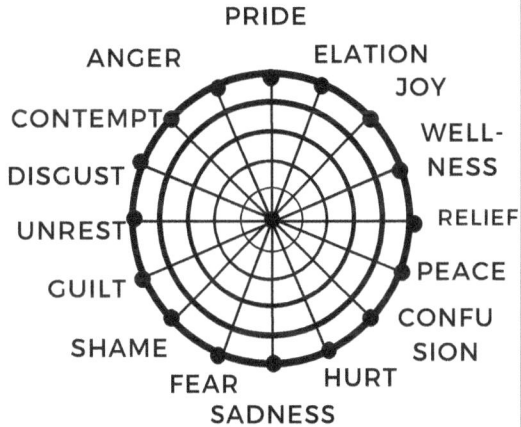

PRIDE
ANGER   ELATION
                JOY
CONTEMPT
                WELL-
DISGUST   NESS
                RELIEF
UNREST
                PEACE
GUILT   CONFU
                SION
SHAME
        FEAR   HURT
        SADNESS

Things to celebrate ......

_____
_____
_____
_____
_____

NEXT APPOINTMENT DATE & TIME

Check in

Doctor's APPOINTMENT

DATE _____

HOW AM I FEELING TODAY?

☐ ☐ ☐ ☐ ☐ ☐ ☐ ☐ ☐ ☐

NOT GREAT   INCREDIBLE

Doctor's name & info

REASON FOR VISIT

_____
_____
_____
_____
_____
_____

INSTRUCTIONS GUIDE

_____
_____
_____
_____

NEXT STEPS

_____
_____
_____
_____
_____

RESULTS

_____
_____
_____
_____
_____

EMOTIONAL WHEEL

PRIDE
ANGER   ELATION
                JOY
CONTEMPT
                WELL-
                NESS
DISGUST
                RELIEF
UNREST
                PEACE
GUILT   CONFU
                SION
SHAME
        HURT
    FEAR
    SADNESS

Things to celebrate......

_____
_____
_____
_____
_____

NEXT APPOINTMENT DATE & TIME

Check in

Doctor's APPOINTMENT   DATE _____

HOW AM I FEELING TODAY?

☐ ☐ ☐ ☐ ☐ ☐ ☐ ☐ ☐ ☐

NOT GREAT   INCREDIBLE

Doctor's name & info

REASON FOR VISIT

_____
_____
_____
_____
_____

INSTRUCTIONS GUIDE

_____
_____
_____
_____

RESULTS

_____
_____
_____
_____
_____

EMOTIONAL WHEEL

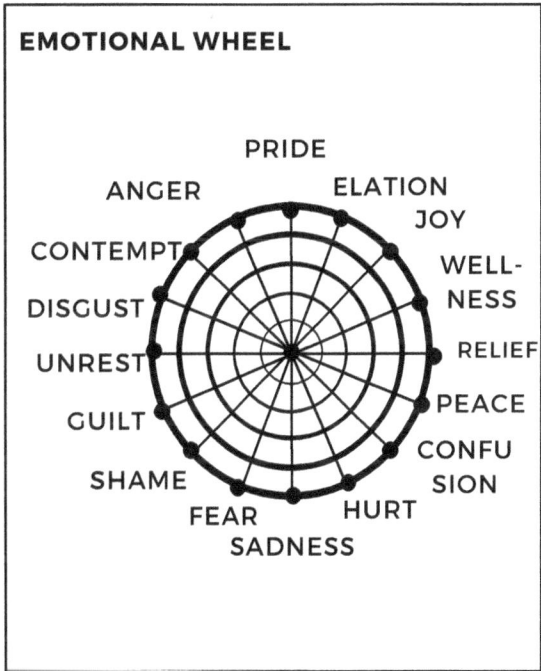

PRIDE

ANGER   ELATION

JOY

CONTEMPT

WELL-NESS

DISGUST

RELIEF

UNREST

PEACE

GUILT

CONFU SION

SHAME

SADNESS   HURT

FEAR

NEXT STEPS

_____
_____
_____
_____
_____

Things to celebrate......

_____
_____
_____
_____

NEXT APPOINTMENT DATE & TIME

Check in

Doctor's APPOINTMENT

DATE _____

HOW AM I FEELING TODAY?

☐ ☐ ☐ ☐ ☐ ☐ ☐ ☐ ☐ ☐

NOT GREAT   INCREDIBLE

Doctor's name &
info

RESULTS

_____
_____
_____
_____
_____
_____

REASON FOR VISIT

_____
_____
_____
_____
_____
_____

EMOTIONAL WHEEL

PRIDE
ANGER   ELATION
                        JOY
CONTEMPT
                    WELL-
                    NESS
DISGUST
                        RELIEF
UNREST
                    PEACE
GUILT
                    CONFU
SHAME   SION
        FEAR   HURT
        SADNESS

INSTRUCTIONS GUIDE

_____
_____
_____
_____

NEXT STEPS

_____
_____
_____
_____
_____

Things to celebrate......

_____
_____
_____
_____
_____

NEXT APPOINTMENT DATE & TIME

Check in

Doctor's APPOINTMENT   DATE _____

HOW AM I FEELING TODAY?

☐ ☐ ☐ ☐ ☐ ☐ ☐ ☐ ☐ ☐

NOT GREAT   INCREDIBLE

Doctor's name & info

REASON FOR VISIT

_____
_____
_____
_____
_____
_____

INSTRUCTIONS GUIDE

_____
_____
_____
_____

RESULTS

_____
_____
_____
_____
_____

EMOTIONAL WHEEL

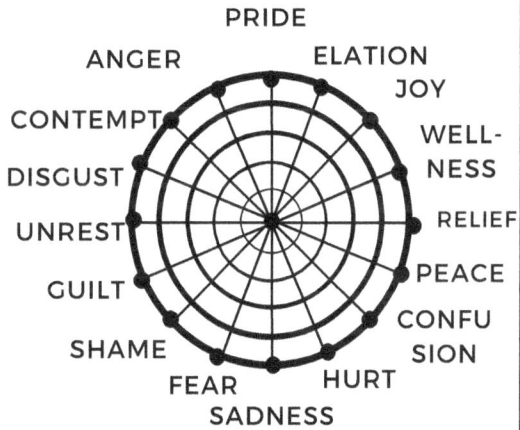

PRIDE
ANGER   ELATION
                    JOY
CONTEMPT
                    WELL-
DISGUST   NESS
UNREST   RELIEF
                    PEACE
GUILT   CONFU
                    SION
SHAME
      FEAR   HURT
      SADNESS

NEXT STEPS

_____
_____
_____
_____
_____

Things to celebrate......

_____
_____
_____
_____
_____

NEXT APPOINTMENT DATE & TIME

Check in

Doctor's APPOINTMENT   DATE _____

HOW AM I FEELING TODAY?

☐ ☐ ☐ ☐ ☐ ☐ ☐ ☐ ☐ ☐

NOT GREAT   INCREDIBLE

Doctor's name & info

REASON FOR VISIT

_____
_____
_____
_____
_____
_____

INSTRUCTIONS GUIDE

_____
_____
_____
_____

RESULTS

_____
_____
_____
_____
_____
_____

EMOTIONAL WHEEL

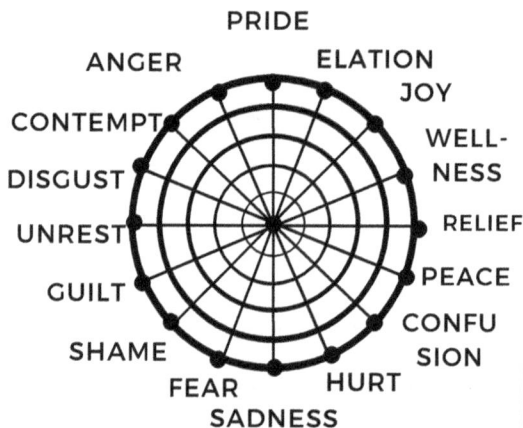

PRIDE
ANGER   ELATION
                JOY
CONTEMPT
                WELL-
DISGUST   NESS
UNREST   RELIEF
GUILT   PEACE
                CONFU
SHAME   SION
    FEAR   HURT
    SADNESS

NEXT STEPS

_____
_____
_____
_____
_____

Things to celebrate......

_____
_____
_____
_____
_____

NEXT APPOINTMENT DATE & TIME

Check in

Doctor's APPOINTMENT   DATE _____

HOW AM I FEELING TODAY?

☐ ☐ ☐ ☐ ☐ ☐ ☐ ☐ ☐ ☐

NOT GREAT   INCREDIBLE

Doctor's name &
info

REASON FOR VISIT

_____

_____

_____

_____

_____

INSTRUCTIONS GUIDE

_____

_____

_____

_____

NEXT STEPS

_____

_____

_____

_____

_____

RESULTS

_____

_____

_____

_____

_____

EMOTIONAL WHEEL

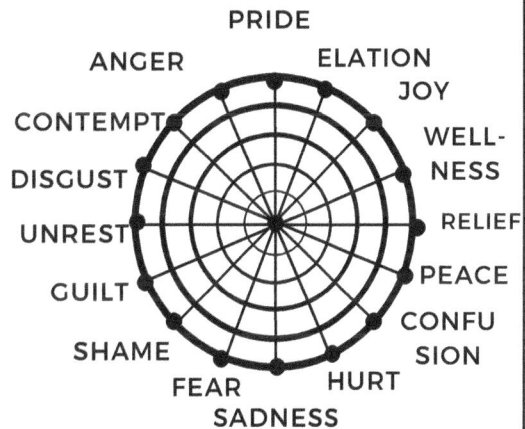

PRIDE

ANGER   ELATION

                         JOY

CONTEMPT

                         WELL-
DISGUST   NESS

UNREST   RELIEF

                      PEACE

GUILT   CONFU
                   SION
SHAME

       FEAR   HURT
       SADNESS

Things to celebrate......

_____

_____

_____

_____

_____

NEXT APPOINTMENT DATE & TIME

Check in

Doctor's APPOINTMENT   DATE _____

HOW AM I FEELING TODAY?

☐ ☐ ☐ ☐ ☐ ☐ ☐ ☐ ☐ ☐

NOT GREAT   INCREDIBLE

Doctor's name &
info

REASON FOR VISIT

_____
_____
_____
_____
_____

INSTRUCTIONS GUIDE

_____
_____
_____
_____

RESULTS

_____
_____
_____
_____
_____

EMOTIONAL WHEEL

PRIDE

ANGER   ELATION

JOY

CONTEMPT   WELL-
NESS

DISGUST

RELIEF

UNREST

PEACE

GUILT   CONFU
SION

SHAME   HURT

FEAR
SADNESS

NEXT STEPS

_____
_____
_____
_____
_____

Things to celebrate......

_____
_____
_____
_____
_____

NEXT APPOINTMENT DATE & TIME

Check in

Doctor's APPOINTMENT DATE _____

HOW AM I FEELING TODAY?

☐ ☐ ☐ ☐ ☐ ☐ ☐ ☐ ☐ ☐

NOT GREAT   INCREDIBLE

Doctor's name & info

REASON FOR VISIT

_____
_____
_____
_____
_____

INSTRUCTIONS GUIDE

_____
_____
_____
_____

RESULTS

_____
_____
_____
_____
_____
_____

EMOTIONAL WHEEL

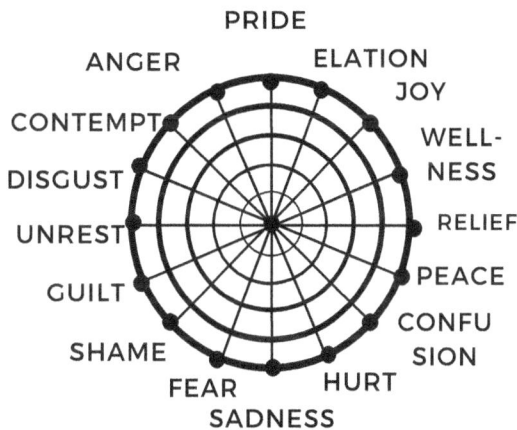

PRIDE
ANGER ELATION
JOY
CONTEMPT
WELL-NESS
DISGUST
RELIEF
UNREST
PEACE
GUILT CONFU SION
SHAME HURT
FEAR
SADNESS

NEXT STEPS

_____
_____
_____
_____
_____

Things to celebrate......

_____
_____
_____
_____

NEXT APPOINTMENT DATE & TIME

Check in

Doctor's APPOINTMENT   DATE _____

HOW AM I FEELING TODAY?

☐ ☐ ☐ ☐ ☐ ☐ ☐ ☐ ☐ ☐

NOT GREAT   INCREDIBLE

Doctor's name & info

REASON FOR VISIT

_____
_____
_____
_____
_____

INSTRUCTIONS GUIDE

_____
_____
_____
_____

NEXT STEPS

_____
_____
_____
_____
_____

RESULTS

_____
_____
_____
_____
_____

EMOTIONAL WHEEL

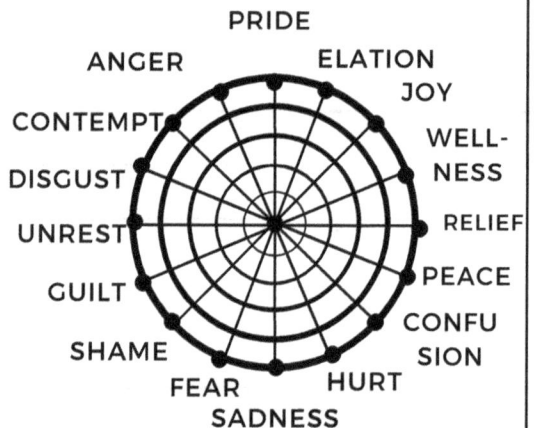

PRIDE
ANGER   ELATION   JOY
CONTEMPT   WELL-NESS
DISGUST   RELIEF
UNREST   PEACE
GUILT   CONFU SION
SHAME   HURT
FEAR   SADNESS

Things to celebrate......

_____
_____
_____
_____

NEXT APPOINTMENT DATE & TIME

Check in

Doctor's APPOINTMENT

DATE _____

HOW AM I FEELING TODAY?

☐ ☐ ☐ ☐ ☐ ☐ ☐ ☐ ☐ ☐

NOT GREAT   INCREDIBLE

Doctor's name & info

REASON FOR VISIT

_____

_____

_____

_____

_____

INSTRUCTIONS GUIDE

_____

_____

_____

_____

NEXT STEPS

_____

_____

_____

_____

_____

RESULTS

_____

_____

_____

_____

_____

EMOTIONAL WHEEL

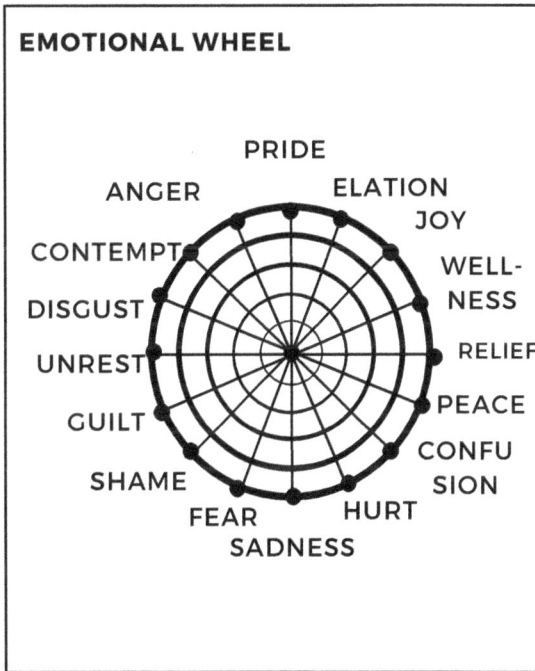

PRIDE
ANGER   ELATION
                JOY
CONTEMPT
                WELL-
DISGUST   NESS
                RELIEF
UNREST
                PEACE
GUILT
                CONFU
SHAME   SION
        FEAR   HURT
        SADNESS

Things to celebrate......

_____

_____

_____

_____

NEXT APPOINTMENT DATE & TIME

Check in

Doctor's APPOINTMENT   DATE _____

HOW AM I FEELING TODAY?

☐ ☐ ☐ ☐ ☐ ☐ ☐ ☐ ☐ ☐

NOT GREAT   INCREDIBLE

Doctor's name & info

REASON FOR VISIT

_____
_____
_____
_____
_____
_____

INSTRUCTIONS GUIDE

_____
_____
_____
_____

NEXT STEPS

_____
_____
_____
_____
_____

RESULTS

_____
_____
_____
_____
_____
_____

EMOTIONAL WHEEL

PRIDE

ANGER   ELATION

JOY

CONTEMPT   WELL-
                      NESS

DISGUST

UNREST   RELIEF

                      PEACE

GUILT   CONFU
                 SION

SHAME   HURT

FEAR

SADNESS

Things to celebrate......

_____
_____
_____
_____
_____

NEXT APPOINTMENT DATE & TIME

Check in

Doctor's APPOINTMENT DATE _____

HOW AM I FEELING TODAY?

☐ ☐ ☐ ☐ ☐ ☐ ☐ ☐ ☐ ☐

NOT GREAT   INCREDIBLE

Doctor's name &
info

REASON FOR VISIT

_____

_____

_____

_____

_____

INSTRUCTIONS GUIDE

_____

_____

_____

_____

RESULTS

_____

_____

_____

_____

_____

EMOTIONAL WHEEL

PRIDE

ANGER   ELATION
                JOY

CONTEMPT   WELL-
                NESS

DISGUST

UNREST   RELIEF

GUILT   PEACE

SHAME   CONFU
                SION

FEAR   HURT
SADNESS

NEXT STEPS

_____

_____

_____

_____

_____

Things to celebrate......

_____

_____

_____

_____

NEXT APPOINTMENT DATE & TIME

Check in

Doctor's APPOINTMENT DATE _____

HOW AM I FEELING TODAY?

☐ ☐ ☐ ☐ ☐ ☐ ☐ ☐ ☐ ☐

NOT GREAT   INCREDIBLE

Doctor's name & info

REASON FOR VISIT

_____
_____
_____
_____
_____

INSTRUCTIONS GUIDE

_____
_____
_____
_____

NEXT STEPS

_____
_____
_____
_____
_____

RESULTS

_____
_____
_____
_____
_____

EMOTIONAL WHEEL

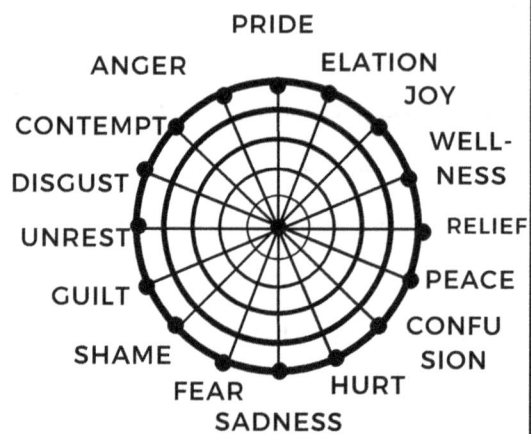

PRIDE
ANGER   ELATION
                JOY
CONTEMPT
                WELL-
DISGUST   NESS
UNREST   RELIEF
                PEACE
GUILT   CONFU
SHAME   SION
        FEAR   HURT
        SADNESS

Things to celebrate......

_____
_____
_____
_____
_____

NEXT APPOINTMENT DATE & TIME

Check in

Doctor's APPOINTMENT

DATE _____

HOW AM I FEELING TODAY?

☐ ☐ ☐ ☐ ☐ ☐ ☐ ☐ ☐ ☐

NOT GREAT   INCREDIBLE

Doctor's name &
info

REASON FOR VISIT

_____
_____
_____
_____
_____
_____

INSTRUCTIONS GUIDE

_____
_____
_____
_____

NEXT STEPS

_____
_____
_____
_____
_____

RESULTS

_____
_____
_____
_____
_____
_____

EMOTIONAL WHEEL

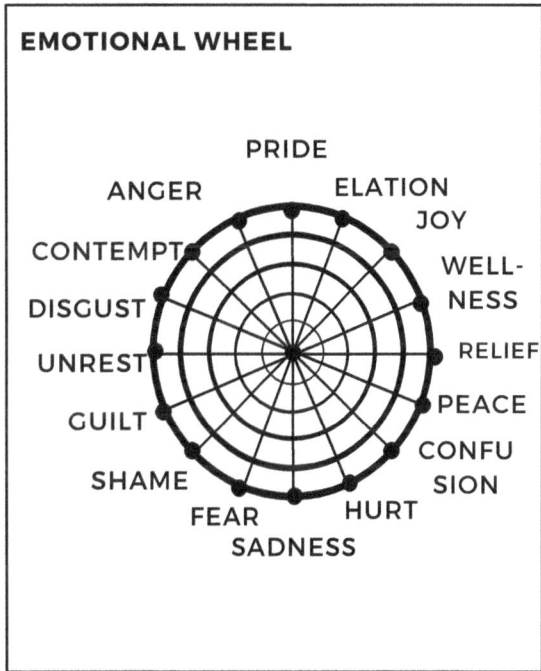

PRIDE
ANGER
ELATION
JOY
CONTEMPT
WELL-NESS
DISGUST
UNREST
RELIEF
PEACE
GUILT
CONFU SION
SHAME
HURT
FEAR
SADNESS

Things to celebrate......

_____
_____
_____
_____
_____

NEXT APPOINTMENT DATE & TIME

Check in

Doctor's APPOINTMENT   DATE _____

HOW AM I FEELING TODAY?

☐ ☐ ☐ ☐ ☐ ☐ ☐ ☐ ☐

NOT GREAT   INCREDIBLE

Doctor's name & info

REASON FOR VISIT

_____

_____

_____

_____

_____

INSTRUCTIONS GUIDE

_____

_____

_____

_____

RESULTS

_____

_____

_____

_____

_____

EMOTIONAL WHEEL

PRIDE
ANGER   ELATION
                    JOY
CONTEMPT
                WELL-
DISGUST   NESS
UNREST   RELIEF
                PEACE
GUILT   CONFU
                SION
SHAME
    FEAR   HURT
    SADNESS

NEXT STEPS

_____

_____

_____

_____

_____

Things to celebrate......

_____

_____

_____

_____

_____

NEXT APPOINTMENT DATE & TIME

Check in

Doctor's APPOINTMENT   DATE _____

HOW AM I FEELING TODAY?

☐ ☐ ☐ ☐ ☐ ☐ ☐ ☐ ☐ ☐

NOT GREAT   INCREDIBLE

Doctor's name & info

REASON FOR VISIT

_____

_____

_____

_____

_____

INSTRUCTIONS GUIDE

_____

_____

_____

_____

NEXT STEPS

_____

_____

_____

_____

_____

RESULTS

_____

_____

_____

_____

_____

EMOTIONAL WHEEL

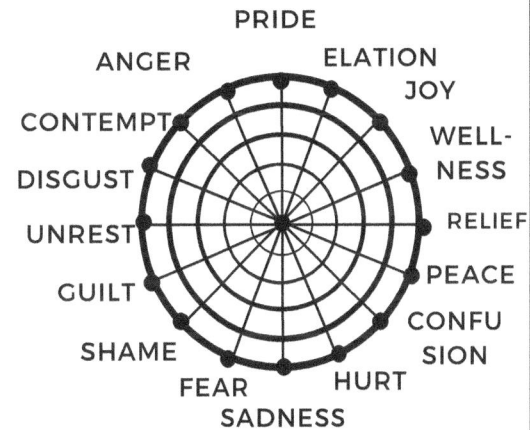

PRIDE

ANGER   ELATION

                        JOY

CONTEMPT   WELL-
                             NESS
DISGUST

UNREST   RELIEF

GUILT   PEACE

                        CONFU
SHAME   SION

     FEAR   HURT
       SADNESS

Things to celebrate......

_____

_____

_____

_____

_____

NEXT APPOINTMENT DATE & TIME

Check in

Doctor's APPOINTMENT   DATE _____

HOW AM I FEELING TODAY?

☐ ☐ ☐ ☐ ☐ ☐ ☐ ☐ ☐ ☐

NOT GREAT   INCREDIBLE

Doctor's name & info

REASON FOR VISIT

_____
_____
_____
_____
_____

INSTRUCTIONS GUIDE

_____
_____
_____
_____

RESULTS

_____
_____
_____
_____
_____

EMOTIONAL WHEEL

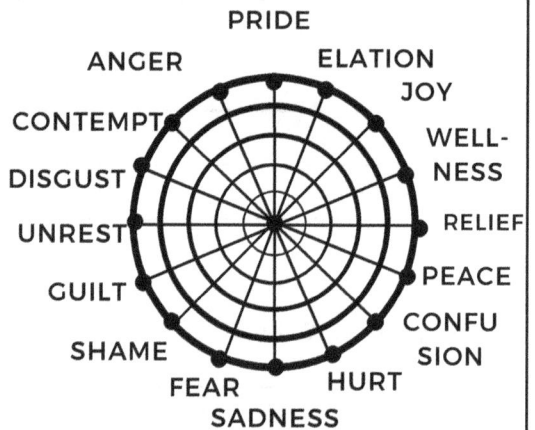

PRIDE
ANGER   ELATION
JOY
CONTEMPT
WELL-NESS
DISGUST
RELIEF
UNREST
PEACE
GUILT
CONFU SION
SHAME
SADNESS HURT
FEAR

NEXT STEPS

_____
_____
_____
_____

Things to celebrate......

_____
_____
_____
_____

NEXT APPOINTMENT DATE & TIME

Check in

Doctor's APPOINTMENT   DATE _____

HOW AM I FEELING TODAY?

☐ ☐ ☐ ☐ ☐ ☐ ☐ ☐ ☐ ☐

NOT GREAT   INCREDIBLE

Doctor's name & info

REASON FOR VISIT

_____
_____
_____
_____
_____
_____

INSTRUCTIONS GUIDE

_____
_____
_____
_____

RESULTS

_____
_____
_____
_____
_____

EMOTIONAL WHEEL

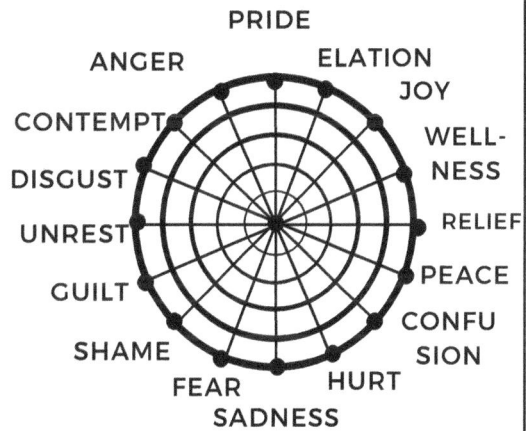

PRIDE

ANGER   ELATION
                          JOY
CONTEMPT
                    WELL-
DISGUST   NESS

UNREST   RELIEF

GUILT   PEACE
                    CONFU
SHAME   SION
        FEAR   HURT
      SADNESS

NEXT STEPS

_____
_____
_____
_____
_____

Things to celebrate......

_____
_____
_____
_____

NEXT APPOINTMENT DATE & TIME

Check in

Doctor's APPOINTMENT DATE _____

HOW AM I FEELING TODAY?

☐ ☐ ☐ ☐ ☐ ☐ ☐ ☐ ☐ ☐

NOT GREAT   INCREDIBLE

Doctor's name & info

REASON FOR VISIT

_____
_____
_____
_____
_____
_____

INSTRUCTIONS GUIDE

_____
_____
_____
_____

RESULTS

_____
_____
_____
_____
_____
_____

EMOTIONAL WHEEL

PRIDE

ANGER   ELATION

     JOY

CONTEMPT

    WELL-NESS

DISGUST

UNREST   RELIEF

    PEACE

GUILT

   CONFU SION

SHAME

FEAR   HURT

SADNESS

NEXT STEPS

_____
_____
_____
_____
_____

Things to celebrate......

_____
_____
_____
_____
_____

NEXT APPOINTMENT DATE & TIME

Check in

Doctor's APPOINTMENT   DATE _____

HOW AM I FEELING TODAY?

☐ ☐ ☐ ☐ ☐ ☐ ☐ ☐ ☐ ☐

NOT GREAT   INCREDIBLE

Doctor's name & info

REASON FOR VISIT

_____

_____

_____

_____

_____

INSTRUCTIONS GUIDE

_____

_____

_____

_____

NEXT STEPS

_____

_____

_____

_____

_____

RESULTS

_____

_____

_____

_____

_____

EMOTIONAL WHEEL

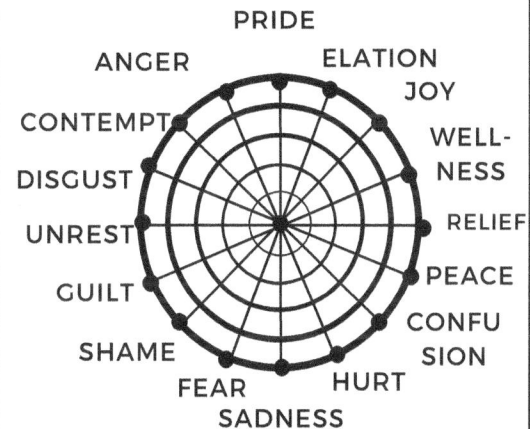

PRIDE

ANGER   ELATION

                    JOY

CONTEMPT   WELL-
                         NESS

DISGUST

UNREST   RELIEF

GUILT   PEACE

                  CONFU
SHAME   SION

   FEAR   HURT
     SADNESS

Things to celebrate ......

_____

_____

_____

_____

NEXT APPOINTMENT DATE & TIME

Check in

Doctor's APPOINTMENT   DATE _____

HOW AM I FEELING TODAY?

☐ ☐ ☐ ☐ ☐ ☐ ☐ ☐ ☐ ☐

NOT GREAT   INCREDIBLE

Doctor's name & info

REASON FOR VISIT

_____
_____
_____
_____
_____
_____

INSTRUCTIONS GUIDE

_____
_____
_____
_____

RESULTS

_____
_____
_____
_____
_____

EMOTIONAL WHEEL

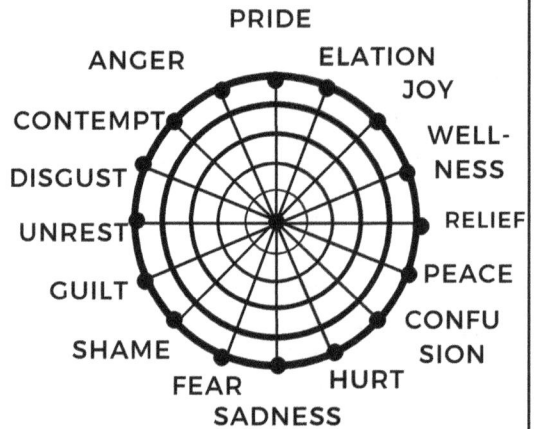

PRIDE
ANGER   ELATION
     JOY
CONTEMPT
     WELL-NESS
DISGUST
UNREST   RELIEF
     PEACE
GUILT   CONFU SION
SHAME
     HURT
FEAR
SADNESS

NEXT STEPS

_____
_____
_____
_____
_____

Things to celebrate ......

_____
_____
_____
_____
_____

NEXT APPOINTMENT DATE & TIME

Check in

Doctor's APPOINTMENT   DATE _____

HOW AM I FEELING TODAY?

☐ ☐ ☐ ☐ ☐ ☐ ☐ ☐ ☐ ☐

NOT GREAT   INCREDIBLE

Doctor's name & info

REASON FOR VISIT

_____

_____

_____

_____

_____

INSTRUCTIONS GUIDE

_____

_____

_____

_____

NEXT STEPS

_____

_____

_____

_____

_____

RESULTS

_____

_____

_____

_____

_____

_____

EMOTIONAL WHEEL

PRIDE
ANGER   ELATION
            JOY
CONTEMPT   WELL-
             NESS
DISGUST
            RELIEF
UNREST
            PEACE
GUILT   CONFU
             SION
SHAME
            HURT
FEAR
SADNESS

Things to celebrate......

_____

_____

_____

_____

NEXT APPOINTMENT DATE & TIME

Check in

Doctor's APPOINTMENT   DATE _____

HOW AM I FEELING TODAY?

☐ ☐ ☐ ☐ ☐ ☐ ☐ ☐ ☐

NOT GREAT   INCREDIBLE

Doctor's name & info

REASON FOR VISIT

_____
_____
_____
_____
_____

INSTRUCTIONS GUIDE

_____
_____
_____
_____

RESULTS

_____
_____
_____
_____
_____

EMOTIONAL WHEEL

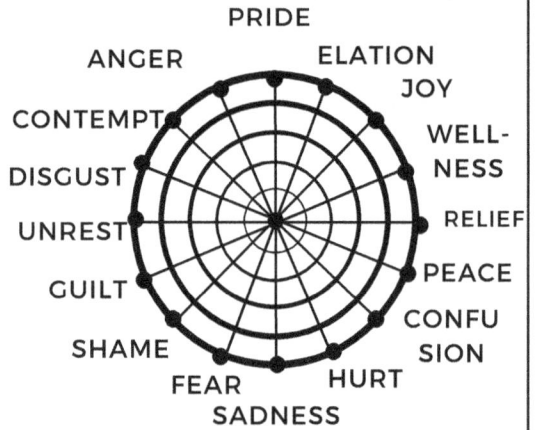

PRIDE
ANGER   ELATION
                    JOY
CONTEMPT
                WELL-
DISGUST   NESS
                RELIEF
UNREST
                PEACE
GUILT   CONFU
                SION
SHAME
        FEAR   HURT
        SADNESS

NEXT STEPS

_____
_____
_____
_____
_____

Things to celebrate......

_____
_____
_____
_____
_____

NEXT APPOINTMENT DATE & TIME

Check in

Doctor's APPOINTMENT   DATE _____

HOW AM I FEELING TODAY?

☐ ☐ ☐ ☐ ☐ ☐ ☐ ☐ ☐

NOT GREAT   INCREDIBLE

Doctor's name &
info

REASON FOR VISIT

_____

_____

_____

_____

_____

INSTRUCTIONS GUIDE

_____

_____

_____

_____

NEXT STEPS

_____

_____

_____

_____

_____

RESULTS

_____

_____

_____

_____

_____

_____

EMOTIONAL WHEEL

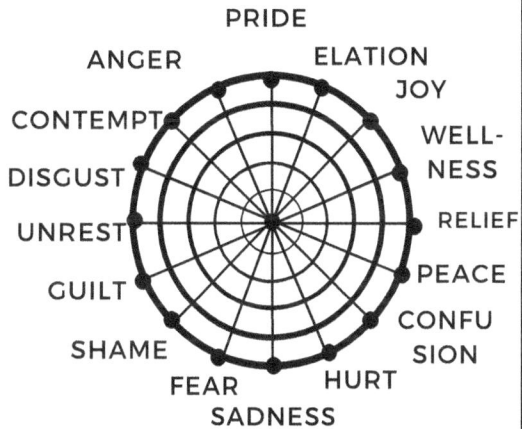

PRIDE
ANGER   ELATION
                    JOY
CONTEMPT   WELL-
                    NESS
DISGUST   RELIEF
UNREST   PEACE
GUILT   CONFU
              SION
SHAME   HURT
    FEAR
    SADNESS

Things to celebrate......

_____

_____

_____

_____

NEXT APPOINTMENT DATE & TIME

Check in

Doctor's APPOINTMENT   DATE _____

HOW AM I FEELING TODAY?

☐ ☐ ☐ ☐ ☐ ☐ ☐ ☐ ☐ ☐

NOT GREAT   INCREDIBLE

Doctor's name & info

REASON FOR VISIT

_____
_____
_____
_____
_____
_____

INSTRUCTIONS GUIDE

_____
_____
_____
_____

RESULTS

_____
_____
_____
_____
_____

EMOTIONAL WHEEL

PRIDE
ANGER   ELATION
                JOY
CONTEMPT
                WELL-
DISGUST   NESS
                RELIEF
UNREST
                PEACE
GUILT   CONFU
                SION
SHAME
        FEAR   HURT
        SADNESS

NEXT STEPS

_____
_____
_____
_____
_____

Things to celebrate ......

_____
_____
_____
_____
_____

NEXT APPOINTMENT DATE & TIME

Check in

Doctor's APPOINTMENT   DATE _____

HOW AM I FEELING TODAY?

☐ ☐ ☐ ☐ ☐ ☐ ☐ ☐ ☐ ☐

NOT GREAT   INCREDIBLE

Doctor's name & info

REASON FOR VISIT

_____

_____

_____

_____

_____

INSTRUCTIONS GUIDE

_____

_____

_____

_____

NEXT STEPS

_____

_____

_____

_____

_____

RESULTS

_____

_____

_____

_____

_____

EMOTIONAL WHEEL

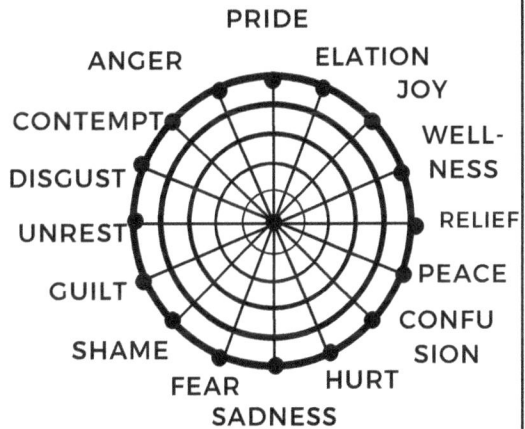

PRIDE

ANGER   ELATION

JOY

CONTEMPT   WELL-
NESS

DISGUST

RELIEF

UNREST

PEACE

GUILT

CONFU
SION

SHAME   HURT

FEAR

SADNESS

Things to celebrate......

_____

_____

_____

_____

NEXT APPOINTMENT DATE & TIME

175

Check in

Doctor's APPOINTMENT   DATE _____

HOW AM I FEELING TODAY?

☐ ☐ ☐ ☐ ☐ ☐ ☐ ☐ ☐

NOT GREAT   INCREDIBLE

Doctor's name & info

REASON FOR VISIT

_____
_____
_____
_____
_____

INSTRUCTIONS GUIDE

_____
_____
_____
_____

RESULTS

_____
_____
_____
_____
_____

EMOTIONAL WHEEL

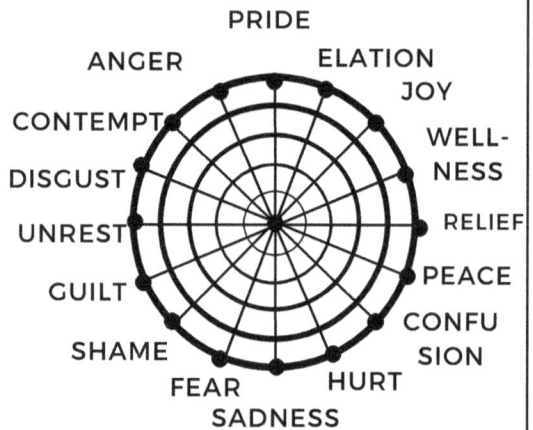

PRIDE
ANGER   ELATION
      JOY
CONTEMPT
      WELL-NESS
DISGUST
      RELIEF
UNREST
      PEACE
GUILT
      CONFUSION
SHAME   HURT
FEAR
SADNESS

NEXT STEPS

_____
_____
_____
_____
_____

Things to celebrate......

_____
_____
_____
_____
_____

NEXT APPOINTMENT DATE & TIME

Check in

Doctor's APPOINTMENT DATE _____

HOW AM I FEELING TODAY?

☐ ☐ ☐ ☐ ☐ ☐ ☐ ☐ ☐

NOT GREAT   INCREDIBLE

Doctor's name & info

REASON FOR VISIT

_____
_____
_____
_____
_____

INSTRUCTIONS GUIDE

_____
_____
_____
_____

RESULTS

_____
_____
_____
_____
_____

EMOTIONAL WHEEL

PRIDE
ANGER   ELATION
                JOY
CONTEMPT   WELL-
DISGUST   NESS
UNREST   RELIEF
GUILT   PEACE
SHAME   CONFU
                SION
FEAR   HURT
SADNESS

NEXT STEPS

_____
_____
_____
_____
_____

Things to celebrate......

_____
_____
_____
_____
_____

NEXT APPOINTMENT DATE & TIME

Check in

Doctor's APPOINTMENT   DATE _____

HOW AM I FEELING TODAY?

☐ ☐ ☐ ☐ ☐ ☐ ☐ ☐ ☐ ☐

NOT GREAT   INCREDIBLE

Doctor's name & info

REASON FOR VISIT

_____
_____
_____
_____
_____

INSTRUCTIONS GUIDE

_____
_____
_____
_____

NEXT STEPS

_____
_____
_____
_____
_____

RESULTS

_____
_____
_____
_____
_____
_____

EMOTIONAL WHEEL

PRIDE
ANGER   ELATION
                    JOY
CONTEMPT
                  WELL-
DISGUST   NESS
UNREST   RELIEF
                  PEACE
GUILT   CONFU
                 SION
SHAME
       FEAR   HURT
       SADNESS

Things to celebrate......

_____
_____
_____
_____
_____

NEXT APPOINTMENT DATE & TIME

Check in

Doctor's APPOINTMENT   DATE _____

HOW AM I FEELING TODAY?

☐ ☐ ☐ ☐ ☐ ☐ ☐ ☐ ☐ ☐

NOT GREAT   INCREDIBLE

Doctor's name & info

REASON FOR VISIT

_____
_____
_____
_____
_____

INSTRUCTIONS GUIDE

_____
_____
_____
_____

NEXT STEPS

_____
_____
_____
_____
_____

RESULTS

_____
_____
_____
_____
_____

EMOTIONAL WHEEL

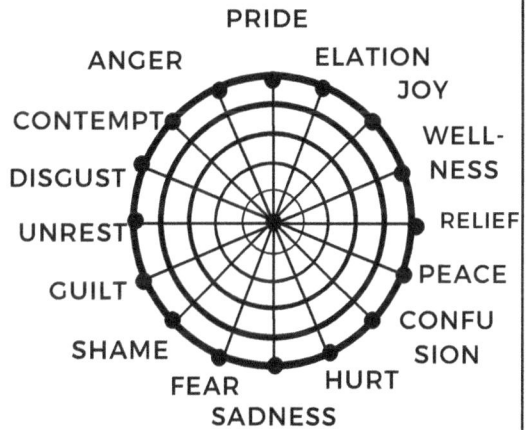

PRIDE
ANGER   ELATION
                JOY
CONTEMPT
                WELL-
                NESS
DISGUST
                RELIEF
UNREST
                PEACE
GUILT
                CONFU
SHAME   SION
        FEAR   HURT
        SADNESS

Things to celebrate......

_____
_____
_____
_____
_____

NEXT APPOINTMENT DATE & TIME

Check in

Doctor's APPOINTMENT   DATE _____

HOW AM I FEELING TODAY?

☐ ☐ ☐ ☐ ☐ ☐ ☐ ☐ ☐

NOT GREAT   INCREDIBLE

Doctor's name &
info

REASON FOR VISIT

_____

_____

_____

_____

_____

_____

INSTRUCTIONS GUIDE

_____

_____

_____

_____

RESULTS

_____

_____

_____

_____

_____

_____

EMOTIONAL WHEEL

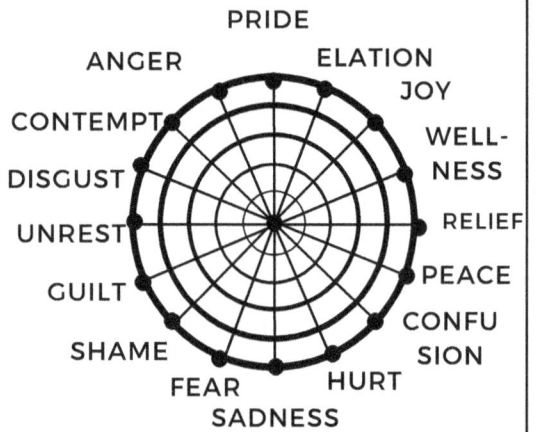

PRIDE

ANGER   ELATION

JOY

CONTEMPT   WELL-
NESS

DISGUST

RELIEF

UNREST

PEACE

GUILT   CONFU
SION

SHAME   HURT

FEAR

SADNESS

NEXT STEPS

_____

_____

_____

_____

_____

Things to celebrate......

_____

_____

_____

_____

_____

NEXT APPOINTMENT DATE & TIME

Check in

Doctor's APPOINTMENT   DATE _____

HOW AM I FEELING TODAY?

☐ ☐ ☐ ☐ ☐ ☐ ☐ ☐ ☐ ☐

NOT GREAT   INCREDIBLE

Doctor's name &
info

REASON FOR VISIT

_____

_____

_____

_____

_____

INSTRUCTIONS GUIDE

_____

_____

_____

_____

NEXT STEPS

_____

_____

_____

_____

_____

RESULTS

_____

_____

_____

_____

_____

EMOTIONAL WHEEL

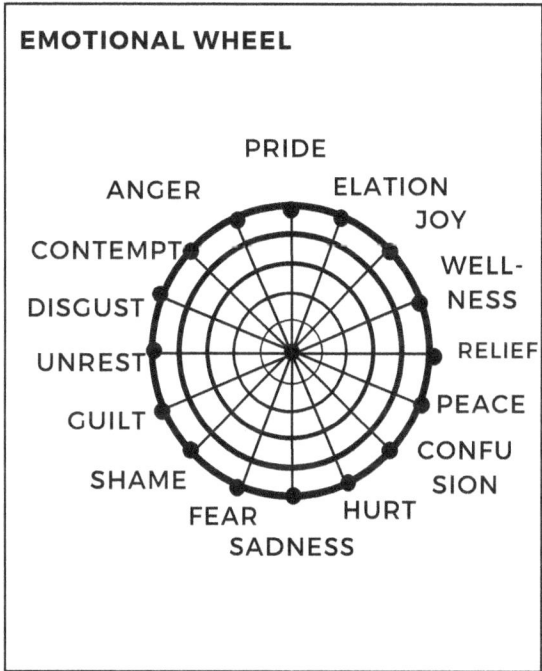

PRIDE

ANGER   ELATION

JOY

CONTEMPT   WELL-
                            NESS

DISGUST

UNREST   RELIEF

                          PEACE

GUILT   CONFU
                           SION

SHAME

FEAR   HURT

SADNESS

Things to celebrate .....

_____

_____

_____

_____

_____

NEXT APPOINTMENT DATE & TIME

Check in

Doctor's APPOINTMENT   DATE _____

HOW AM I FEELING TODAY?

☐ ☐ ☐ ☐ ☐ ☐ ☐ ☐ ☐ ☐

NOT GREAT   INCREDIBLE

Doctor's name & info

REASON FOR VISIT

_____
_____
_____
_____
_____
_____

INSTRUCTIONS GUIDE

_____
_____
_____
_____

NEXT STEPS

_____
_____
_____
_____
_____

RESULTS

_____
_____
_____
_____
_____

EMOTIONAL WHEEL

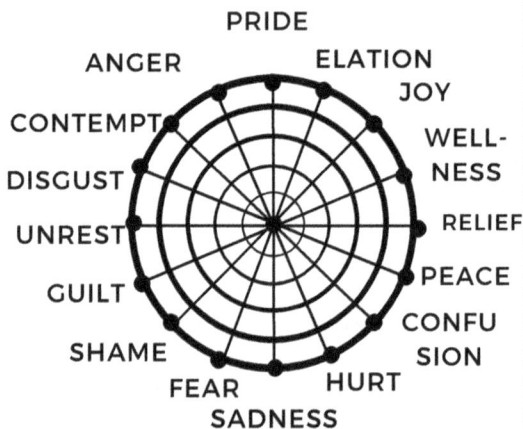

PRIDE
ANGER   ELATION
                    JOY
CONTEMPT
                    WELL-
DISGUST   NESS
                    RELIEF
UNREST
                    PEACE
GUILT   CONFU
SHAME   SION
      FEAR   HURT
      SADNESS

Things to celebrate......

_____
_____
_____
_____
_____

NEXT APPOINTMENT DATE & TIME

Check in

Doctor's APPOINTMENT   DATE _____

HOW AM I FEELING TODAY?

☐ ☐ ☐ ☐ ☐ ☐ ☐ ☐ ☐ ☐

NOT GREAT   INCREDIBLE

Doctor's name & info

REASON FOR VISIT

_____
_____
_____
_____
_____

INSTRUCTIONS GUIDE

_____
_____
_____
_____

NEXT STEPS

_____
_____
_____
_____
_____

RESULTS

_____
_____
_____
_____
_____
_____

EMOTIONAL WHEEL

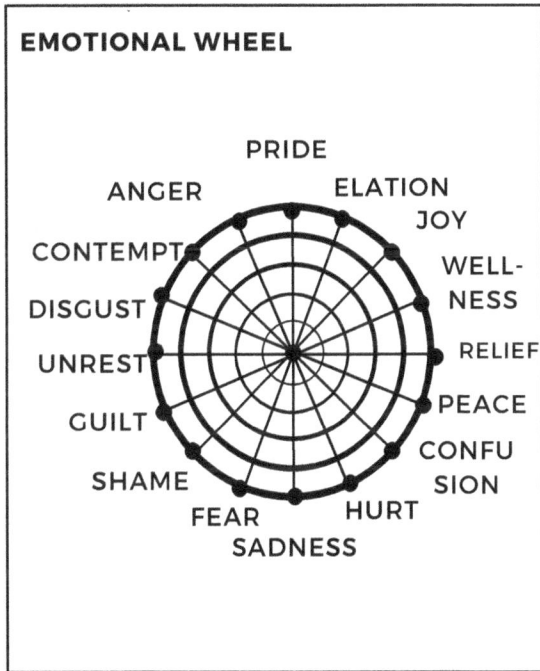

PRIDE

ANGER   ELATION

JOY

CONTEMPT   WELL-
NESS

DISGUST

UNREST   RELIEF

GUILT   PEACE

CONFU
SION

SHAME

FEAR   HURT

SADNESS

Things to celebrate......

_____
_____
_____
_____
_____

NEXT APPOINTMENT DATE & TIME

Check in

Doctor's APPOINTMENT   DATE _____

HOW AM I FEELING TODAY?

☐ ☐ ☐ ☐ ☐ ☐ ☐ ☐ ☐ ☐

NOT GREAT   INCREDIBLE

Doctor's name & info

REASON FOR VISIT

_____
_____
_____
_____
_____

INSTRUCTIONS GUIDE

_____
_____
_____
_____

RESULTS

_____
_____
_____
_____
_____

EMOTIONAL WHEEL

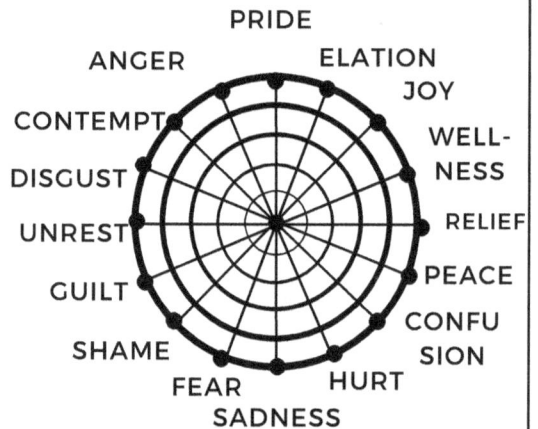

PRIDE
ANGER   ELATION
                  JOY
CONTEMPT
                  WELL-
DISGUST   NESS
UNREST   RELIEF
                  PEACE
GUILT   CONFU
                  SION
SHAME   HURT
      FEAR
      SADNESS

NEXT STEPS

_____
_____
_____
_____
_____

Things to celebrate......

_____
_____
_____
_____
_____

NEXT APPOINTMENT DATE & TIME

Check in

Doctor's APPOINTMENT   DATE _____

HOW AM I FEELING TODAY?

☐ ☐ ☐ ☐ ☐ ☐ ☐ ☐ ☐

NOT GREAT   INCREDIBLE

Doctor's name &
info

REASON FOR VISIT

_____

_____

_____

_____

_____

INSTRUCTIONS GUIDE

_____

_____

_____

_____

RESULTS

_____

_____

_____

_____

_____

_____

EMOTIONAL WHEEL

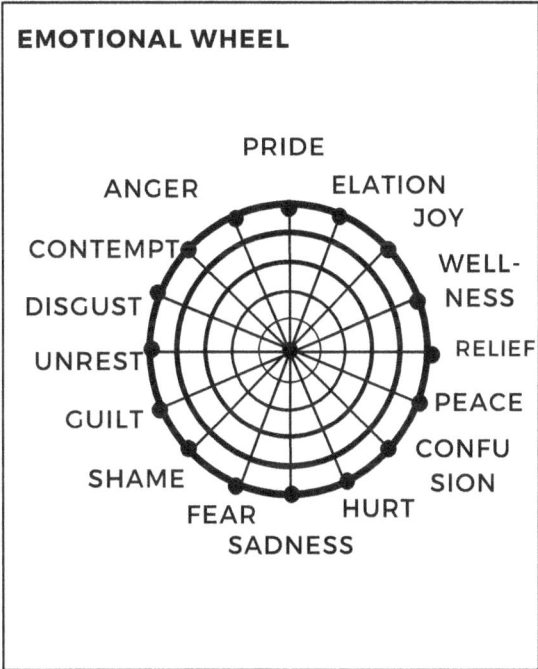

PRIDE
ANGER   ELATION
                    JOY
CONTEMPT   WELL-
                         NESS
DISGUST
                    RELIEF
UNREST
                    PEACE
GUILT   CONFU
                  SION
SHAME
FEAR   HURT
SADNESS

NEXT STEPS

_____

_____

_____

_____

_____

Things to celebrate......

_____

_____

_____

_____

_____

NEXT APPOINTMENT DATE & TIME

Check in

Doctor's APPOINTMENT   DATE _____

HOW AM I FEELING TODAY?

☐ ☐ ☐ ☐ ☐ ☐ ☐ ☐ ☐ ☐

NOT GREAT   INCREDIBLE

Doctor's name & info

REASON FOR VISIT

_____
_____
_____
_____
_____

INSTRUCTIONS GUIDE

_____
_____
_____
_____

RESULTS

_____
_____
_____
_____
_____

EMOTIONAL WHEEL

PRIDE
ANGER   ELATION
                JOY
CONTEMPT
                WELL-
DISGUST   NESS
                RELIEF
UNREST
                PEACE
GUILT   CONFU
SHAME   SION
    FEAR   HURT
    SADNESS

NEXT STEPS

_____
_____
_____
_____
_____

Things to celebrate......

_____
_____
_____
_____
_____

NEXT APPOINTMENT DATE & TIME

Check in

Doctor's APPOINTMENT   DATE _____

HOW AM I FEELING TODAY?

☐ ☐ ☐ ☐ ☐ ☐ ☐ ☐ ☐ ☐

NOT GREAT   INCREDIBLE

Doctor's name & info

REASON FOR VISIT

_____
_____
_____
_____
_____
_____

INSTRUCTIONS GUIDE

_____
_____
_____
_____

NEXT STEPS

_____
_____
_____
_____
_____

RESULTS

_____
_____
_____
_____
_____
_____

EMOTIONAL WHEEL

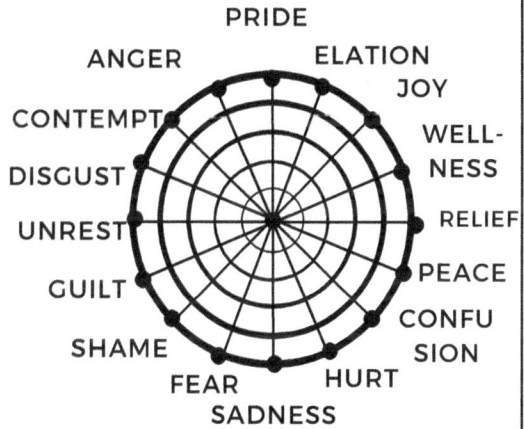

PRIDE

ANGER   ELATION
                JOY
CONTEMPT   WELL-
                 NESS
DISGUST
                RELIEF
UNREST
              PEACE
GUILT   CONFU
              SION
SHAME   HURT
FEAR
SADNESS

Things to celebrate......

_____
_____
_____
_____

NEXT APPOINTMENT DATE & TIME

Check in

Doctor's APPOINTMENT   DATE _____

HOW AM I FEELING TODAY?

☐ ☐ ☐ ☐ ☐ ☐ ☐ ☐ ☐

NOT GREAT   INCREDIBLE

Doctor's name & info

REASON FOR VISIT

_____

_____

_____

_____

_____

INSTRUCTIONS GUIDE

_____

_____

_____

_____

NEXT STEPS

_____

_____

_____

_____

_____

RESULTS

_____

_____

_____

_____

_____

_____

EMOTIONAL WHEEL

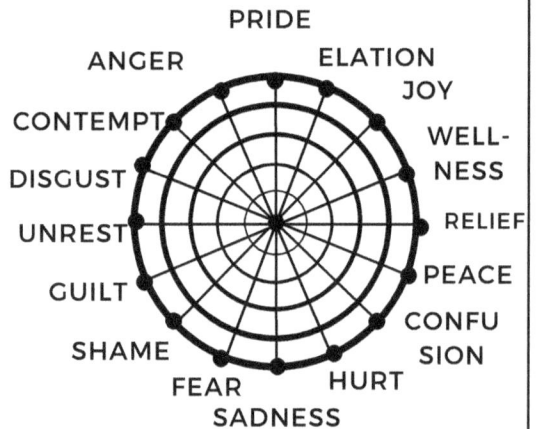

PRIDE
ANGER   ELATION
                JOY
CONTEMPT
            WELL-
DISGUST   NESS
UNREST   RELIEF
GUILT   PEACE
            CONFU
SHAME   SION
    FEAR   HURT
    SADNESS

Things to celebrate......

_____

_____

_____

_____

NEXT APPOINTMENT DATE & TIME

Check in

Doctor's APPOINTMENT   DATE _____

HOW AM I FEELING TODAY?

☐ ☐ ☐ ☐ ☐ ☐ ☐ ☐ ☐

NOT GREAT   INCREDIBLE

*Doctor's name &
info*

REASON FOR VISIT

_____
_____
_____
_____
_____

INSTRUCTIONS GUIDE

_____
_____
_____
_____

RESULTS

_____
_____
_____
_____
_____

EMOTIONAL WHEEL

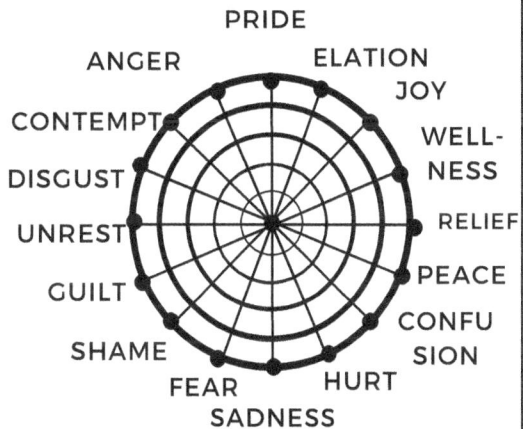

PRIDE

ANGER   ELATION
                     JOY

CONTEMPT   WELL-
                       NESS
DISGUST

UNREST   RELIEF

GUILT   PEACE

                   CONFU
SHAME   SION

      FEAR   HURT
       SADNESS

NEXT STEPS

_____
_____
_____
_____
_____

Things to celebrate ......

_____
_____
_____
_____
_____

NEXT APPOINTMENT DATE & TIME

Check in

Radiation APPOINTMENT   DATE _____

HOW AM I FEELING TODAY?

☐ ☐ ☐ ☐ ☐ ☐ ☐ ☐ ☐ ☐

NOT GREAT   INCREDIBLE

Radiation
Center name &
info

DOS

_____
_____
_____
_____
_____
_____

DON'TS

_____
_____
_____

SIDE EFFECTS

_____
_____
_____
_____
_____

SYMPTOMS

_____
_____
_____
_____
_____

EMOTIONAL WHEEL

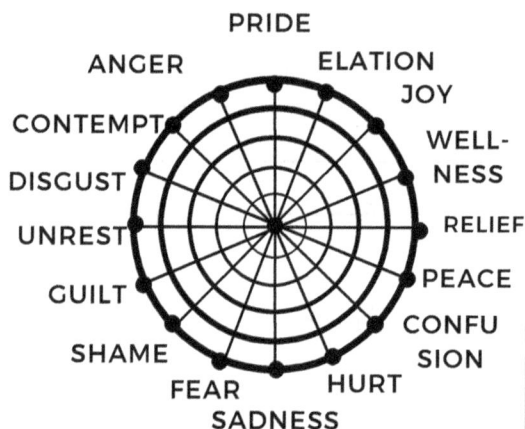

PRIDE
ANGER   ELATION
                JOY
CONTEMPT
                WELL-
DISGUST   NESS
UNREST   RELIEF
GUILT   PEACE
                CONFU
SHAME   SION
      FEAR   HURT
      SADNESS

Things to celebrate ......

_____
_____
_____
_____
_____

NEXT APPOINTMENT DATE & TIME

Check in

Radiation APPOINTMENT   DATE _____

HOW AM I FEELING TODAY?

☐ ☐ ☐ ☐ ☐ ☐ ☐ ☐ ☐ ☐

NOT GREAT   INCREDIBLE

*Radiation
Center name &
info*

SYMPTOMS

_____
_____
_____
_____
_____

DOS

_____
_____
_____
_____
_____

DON'TS

_____
_____
_____

EMOTIONAL WHEEL

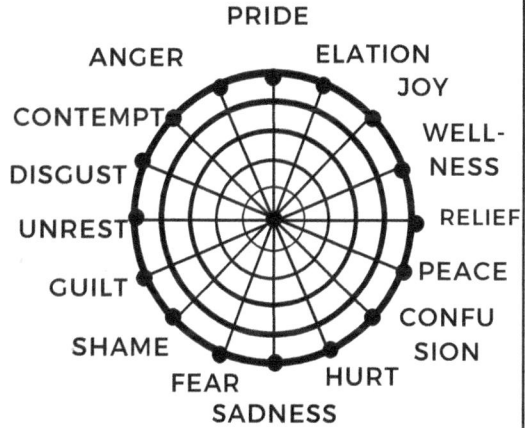

PRIDE
ANGER   ELATION
                    JOY
CONTEMPT
                    WELL-
DISGUST   NESS
UNREST   RELIEF
                    PEACE
GUILT
                 CONFU
SHAME   SION
    FEAR   HURT
      SADNESS

SIDE EFFECTS

_____
_____
_____
_____
_____

Things to celebrate......

_____
_____
_____
_____
_____

NEXT APPOINTMENT DATE & TIME

Check in

Radiation APPOINTMENT   DATE _____

HOW AM I FEELING TODAY?

☐ ☐ ☐ ☐ ☐ ☐ ☐ ☐ ☐ ☐

NOT GREAT   INCREDIBLE

*Radiation
Center name &
info*

DOS

_____
_____
_____
_____
_____
_____

DON'TS

_____
_____
_____
_____

SYMPTOMS

_____
_____
_____
_____
_____

EMOTIONAL WHEEL

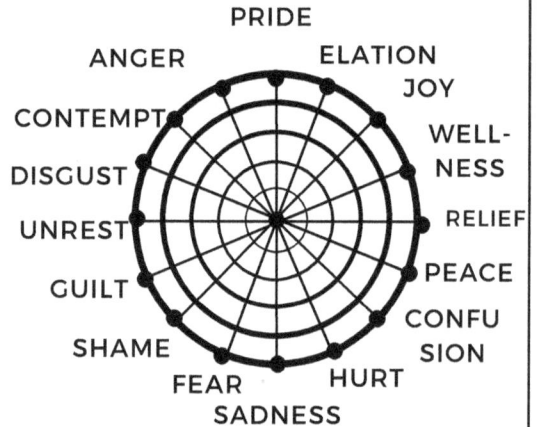

PRIDE
ANGER   ELATION
                              JOY
CONTEMPT
                         WELL-
                         NESS
DISGUST
                         RELIEF
UNREST
                         PEACE
GUILT
                         CONFU
SHAME   SION
      FEAR   HURT
        SADNESS

SIDE EFFECTS

_____
_____
_____
_____
_____

Things to celebrate......

_____
_____
_____
_____
_____

NEXT APPOINTMENT DATE & TIME

Check in

Radiation APPOINTMENT   DATE _____

HOW AM I FEELING TODAY?

☐ ☐ ☐ ☐ ☐ ☐ ☐ ☐ ☐ ☐

NOT GREAT   INCREDIBLE

Radiation Center name & info

DOS

_____
_____
_____
_____
_____
_____

DON'TS

_____
_____
_____

SIDE EFFECTS

_____
_____
_____
_____
_____

SYMPTOMS

_____
_____
_____
_____
_____

EMOTIONAL WHEEL

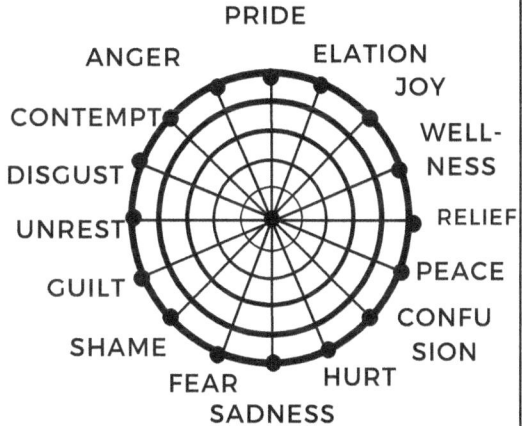

PRIDE
ANGER   ELATION
                JOY
CONTEMPT
             WELL-
DISGUST   NESS

UNREST   RELIEF

GUILT   PEACE

             CONFU
SHAME   SION
        HURT
FEAR
SADNESS

Things to celebrate......

_____
_____
_____
_____
_____

NEXT APPOINTMENT DATE & TIME

Check in

Radiation APPOINTMENT   DATE _____

HOW AM I FEELING TODAY?

☐ ☐ ☐ ☐ ☐ ☐ ☐ ☐ ☐ ☐

NOT GREAT   INCREDIBLE

Radiation
Center name &
info

DOS

_____

_____

_____

_____

_____

DON'TS

_____

_____

_____

SYMPTOMS

_____

_____

_____

_____

_____

EMOTIONAL WHEEL

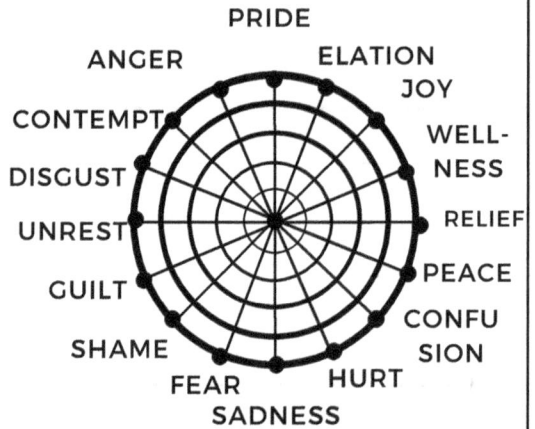

PRIDE
ANGER   ELATION
                JOY
CONTEMPT
                WELL-
DISGUST   NESS
UNREST   RELIEF
GUILT   PEACE
                CONFU
SHAME   SION
    FEAR   HURT
    SADNESS

SIDE EFFECTS

_____

_____

_____

_____

_____

Things to celebrate......

_____

_____

_____

_____

_____

NEXT APPOINTMENT DATE & TIME

Check in

Radiation APPOINTMENT   DATE _____

HOW AM I FEELING TODAY?

☐ ☐ ☐ ☐ ☐ ☐ ☐ ☐ ☐ ☐

NOT GREAT   INCREDIBLE

Radiation
Center name &
info

DOS

_____

_____

_____

_____

_____

DON'TS

_____

_____

_____

SIDE EFFECTS

_____

_____

_____

_____

_____

SYMPTOMS

_____

_____

_____

_____

_____

EMOTIONAL WHEEL

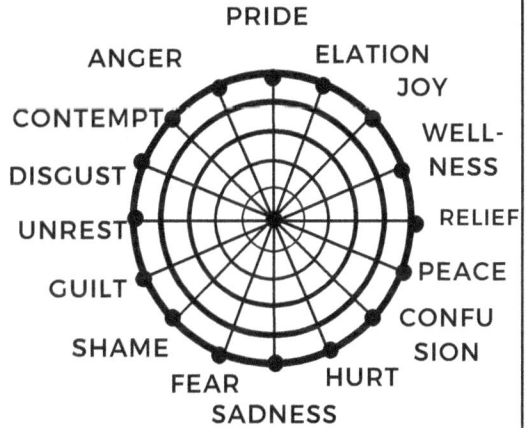

PRIDE
ANGER   ELATION
                JOY
CONTEMPT   WELL-
                NESS
DISGUST
              RELIEF
UNREST
              PEACE
GUILT   CONFU
              SION
SHAME
    FEAR   HURT
    SADNESS

Things to celebrate......

_____

_____

_____

_____

_____

NEXT APPOINTMENT DATE & TIME

Check in

Radiation APPOINTMENT   DATE _____

HOW AM I FEELING TODAY?

☐ ☐ ☐ ☐ ☐ ☐ ☐ ☐ ☐ ☐

NOT GREAT   INCREDIBLE

Radiation
Center name &
info

DOS

_____

_____

_____

_____

_____

DON'TS

_____

_____

_____

_____

SIDE EFFECTS

_____

_____

_____

_____

_____

SYMPTOMS

_____

_____

_____

_____

_____

EMOTIONAL WHEEL

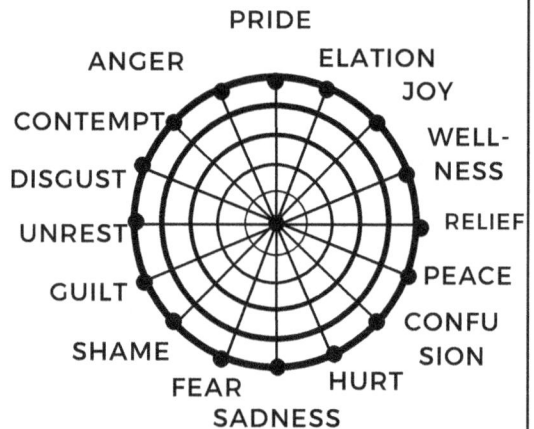

PRIDE
ANGER   ELATION
                    JOY
CONTEMPT
                 WELL-
DISGUST   NESS
UNREST   RELIEF
GUILT   PEACE
                CONFU
SHAME   SION
      FEAR   HURT
      SADNESS

Things to celebrate......

_____

_____

_____

_____

_____

NEXT APPOINTMENT DATE & TIME

Check in

Radiation APPOINTMENT   DATE _____

HOW AM I FEELING TODAY?

☐ ☐ ☐ ☐ ☐ ☐ ☐ ☐ ☐ ☐

NOT GREAT   INCREDIBLE

Radiation Center name & info

DOS

_____

_____

_____

_____

_____

DON'TS

_____

_____

_____

SIDE EFFECTS

_____

_____

_____

_____

_____

SYMPTOMS

_____

_____

_____

_____

_____

EMOTIONAL WHEEL

PRIDE
ANGER   ELATION
                JOY
CONTEMPT
                WELL-
DISGUST   NESS
UNREST   RELIEF
GUILT   PEACE
                CONFU
SHAME   SION
   FEAR   HURT
   SADNESS

Things to celebrate......

_____

_____

_____

_____

_____

NEXT APPOINTMENT DATE & TIME

Check in

Radiation APPOINTMENT   DATE _____

HOW AM I FEELING TODAY?

☐ ☐ ☐ ☐ ☐ ☐ ☐ ☐ ☐ ☐

NOT GREAT   INCREDIBLE

Radiation
Center name &
info

DOS

_____
_____
_____
_____
_____
_____

DON'TS

_____
_____
_____
_____

SIDE EFFECTS

_____
_____
_____
_____
_____

SYMPTOMS

_____
_____
_____
_____
_____

EMOTIONAL WHEEL

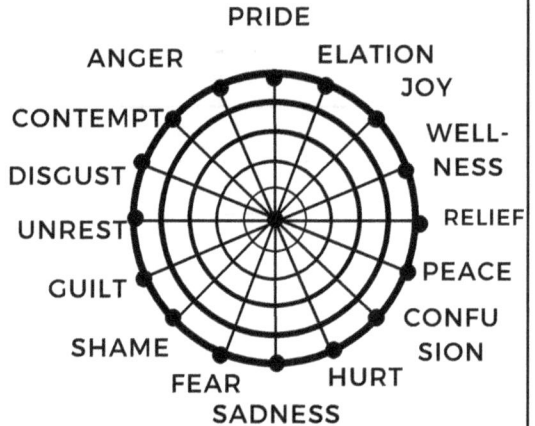

PRIDE
ANGER   ELATION
                      JOY
CONTEMPT
                   WELL-
DISGUST   NESS
                   RELIEF
UNREST
                   PEACE
GUILT   CONFU
                 SION
SHAME
    FEAR   HURT
    SADNESS

Things to celebrate......

_____
_____
_____
_____

NEXT APPOINTMENT DATE & TIME

Check in

Radiation APPOINTMENT   DATE _____

HOW AM I FEELING TODAY?

☐ ☐ ☐ ☐ ☐ ☐ ☐ ☐ ☐ ☐

NOT GREAT   INCREDIBLE

Radiation Center name & info

DOS

_____
_____
_____
_____
_____
_____

DON'TS

_____
_____
_____
_____

SIDE EFFECTS

_____
_____
_____
_____
_____

SYMPTOMS

_____
_____
_____
_____
_____
_____

EMOTIONAL WHEEL

PRIDE
ANGER   ELATION
JOY
CONTEMPT   WELL-NESS
DISGUST   RELIEF
UNREST   PEACE
GUILT   CONFUSION
SHAME   HURT
FEAR
SADNESS

Things to celebrate......

_____
_____
_____
_____
_____

NEXT APPOINTMENT DATE & TIME

Check in

Radiation APPOINTMENT   DATE _____

HOW AM I FEELING TODAY?

☐ ☐ ☐ ☐ ☐ ☐ ☐ ☐ ☐ ☐

NOT GREAT   INCREDIBLE

Radiation Center name & info

DOS

_____

_____

_____

_____

_____

DON'TS

_____

_____

_____

SYMPTOMS

_____

_____

_____

_____

_____

EMOTIONAL WHEEL

PRIDE
ANGER   ELATION
                        JOY
CONTEMPT
                    WELL-
DISGUST   NESS
UNREST   RELIEF
GUILT   PEACE
                    CONFU
SHAME   SION
    FEAR   HURT
    SADNESS

SIDE EFFECTS

_____

_____

_____

_____

_____

Things to celebrate......

_____

_____

_____

_____

NEXT APPOINTMENT DATE & TIME

Check in

Radiation APPOINTMENT   DATE _____

HOW AM I FEELING TODAY?

☐ ☐ ☐ ☐ ☐ ☐ ☐ ☐ ☐ ☐

NOT GREAT   INCREDIBLE

Radiation Center name & info

SYMPTOMS

_____
_____
_____
_____
_____

DOS

_____
_____
_____
_____
_____
_____

DON'TS

_____
_____
_____
_____

EMOTIONAL WHEEL

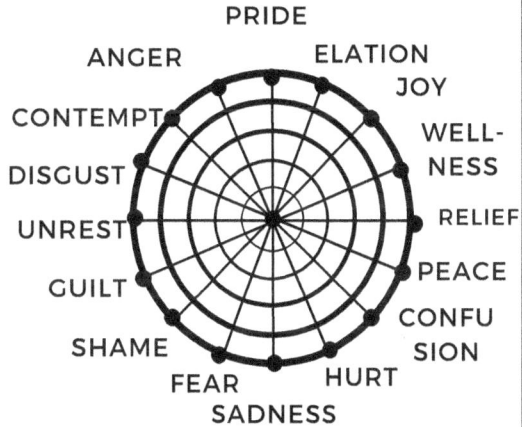

PRIDE
ANGER   ELATION
                    JOY
CONTEMPT   WELL-
                    NESS
DISGUST
                    RELIEF
UNREST
                    PEACE
GUILT
                    CONFU
SHAME   SION
        FEAR   HURT
        SADNESS

SIDE EFFECTS

_____
_____
_____
_____
_____

Things to celebrate......

_____
_____
_____
_____

NEXT APPOINTMENT DATE & TIME

Check in

Chemo APPOINTMENT   DATE _____

HOW AM I FEELING TODAY?

☐ ☐ ☐ ☐ ☐ ☐ ☐ ☐ ☐ ☐

NOT GREAT   INCREDIBLE

C

chemotherapy Center name & info

SYMPTOMS

_____
_____
_____
_____
_____

DOS

_____
_____
_____
_____
_____

DON'TS

_____
_____
_____

EMOTIONAL WHEEL

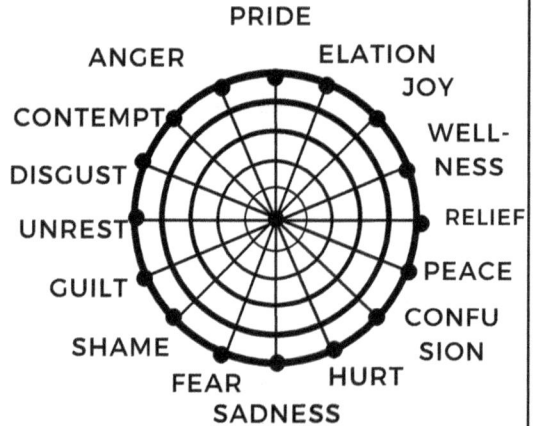

PRIDE
ANGER   ELATION
JOY
CONTEMPT   WELL-NESS
DISGUST
UNREST   RELIEF
GUILT   PEACE
SHAME   CONFU SION
FEAR   HURT
SADNESS

SIDE EFFECTS

_____
_____
_____
_____
_____

Things to celebrate......

_____
_____
_____
_____
_____

NEXT APPOINTMENT DATE & TIME

Check in

Chemo APPOINTMENT DATE _____

HOW AM I FEELING TODAY?

☐ ☐ ☐ ☐ ☐ ☐ ☐ ☐ ☐ ☐

NOT GREAT   INCREDIBLE

Chemotherapy Center name & info

DOS

_____

_____

_____

_____

_____

DON'TS

_____

_____

_____

SIDE EFFECTS

_____

_____

_____

_____

_____

SYMPTOMS

_____

_____

_____

_____

_____

EMOTIONAL WHEEL

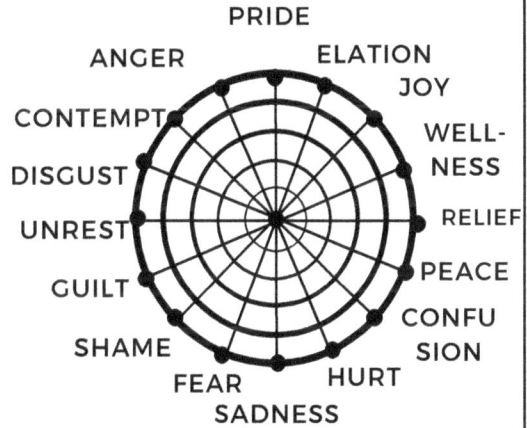

PRIDE
ANGER   ELATION
                    JOY
CONTEMPT
                    WELL-
                    NESS
DISGUST
                    RELIEF
UNREST
                    PEACE
GUILT
                  CONFU
SHAME   SION
        FEAR   HURT
        SADNESS

Things to celebrate......

_____

_____

_____

_____

_____

NEXT APPOINTMENT DATE & TIME

Check in

Chemo APPOINTMENT   DATE _____

HOW AM I FEELING TODAY?

☐ ☐ ☐ ☐ ☐ ☐ ☐ ☐ ☐ ☐

NOT GREAT   INCREDIBLE

*chemotherapy
Center name &
info*

DOS

_____

_____

_____

_____

_____

_____

DON'TS

_____

_____

_____

_____

SYMPTOMS

_____

_____

_____

_____

_____

EMOTIONAL WHEEL

PRIDE

ANGER   ELATION

                              JOY

CONTEMPT   WELL-
                              NESS
DISGUST
                              RELIEF
UNREST
                              PEACE
GUILT
                         CONFU
SHAME   SION

FEAR   HURT
SADNESS

SIDE EFFECTS

_____

_____

_____

_____

_____

Things to celebrate......

_____

_____

_____

_____

NEXT APPOINTMENT DATE & TIME

Check in

Chemo APPOINTMENT   DATE _____

HOW AM I FEELING TODAY?

☐ ☐ ☐ ☐ ☐ ☐ ☐ ☐ ☐ ☐

NOT GREAT   INCREDIBLE

Chemotherapy Center name & info

DOS

_____

_____

_____

_____

_____

_____

DON'TS

_____

_____

_____

_____

SIDE EFFECTS

_____

_____

_____

_____

_____

SYMPTOMS

_____

_____

_____

_____

_____

EMOTIONAL WHEEL

PRIDE
ANGER   ELATION
                    JOY
CONTEMPT   WELL-
                    NESS
DISGUST
UNREST   RELIEF
GUILT   PEACE
              CONFU
SHAME   SION
    FEAR   HURT
    SADNESS

Things to celebrate ......

_____

_____

_____

_____

_____

NEXT APPOINTMENT DATE & TIME

Check in

Chemo APPOINTMENT   DATE _____

HOW AM I FEELING TODAY?

☐ ☐ ☐ ☐ ☐ ☐ ☐ ☐ ☐ ☐

NOT GREAT   INCREDIBLE

*chemotherapy
Center name &
info*

DOS

_____
_____
_____
_____
_____

DON'TS

_____
_____
_____

SYMPTOMS

_____
_____
_____
_____
_____

EMOTIONAL WHEEL

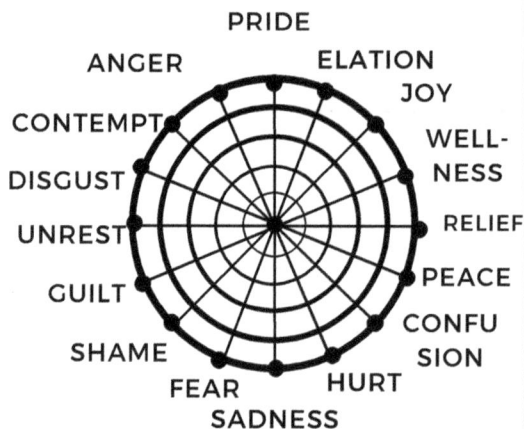

PRIDE
ANGER   ELATION
                JOY
CONTEMPT
                WELL-
DISGUST   NESS
                RELIEF
UNREST
                PEACE
GUILT
            CONFU
SHAME   SION
    FEAR   HURT
    SADNESS

SIDE EFFECTS

_____
_____
_____
_____
_____

Things to celebrate......

_____
_____
_____
_____
_____

NEXT APPOINTMENT DATE & TIME

Check in

Chemo APPOINTMENT   DATE _____

HOW AM I FEELING TODAY?

☐ ☐ ☐ ☐ ☐ ☐ ☐ ☐ ☐ ☐

NOT GREAT   INCREDIBLE

Chemotherapy Center name & info

DOS

_____
_____
_____
_____
_____
_____

DON'TS

_____
_____
_____
_____

SIDE EFFECTS

_____
_____
_____
_____
_____

SYMPTOMS

_____
_____
_____
_____
_____
_____

EMOTIONAL WHEEL

PRIDE
ANGER   ELATION
                        JOY
CONTEMPT
                    WELL-
DISGUST   NESS
UNREST   RELIEF
                    PEACE
GUILT   CONFU
SHAME   SION
   FEAR   HURT
      SADNESS

Things to celebrate......

_____
_____
_____
_____

NEXT APPOINTMENT DATE & TIME

Check in

Chemo APPOINTMENT DATE _____

HOW AM I FEELING TODAY?

☐ ☐ ☐ ☐ ☐ ☐ ☐ ☐ ☐ ☐

NOT GREAT   INCREDIBLE

*chemotherapy
Center name &
info*

SYMPTOMS

_____
_____
_____
_____
_____

DOS

_____
_____
_____
_____
_____

DON'TS

_____
_____
_____
_____

EMOTIONAL WHEEL

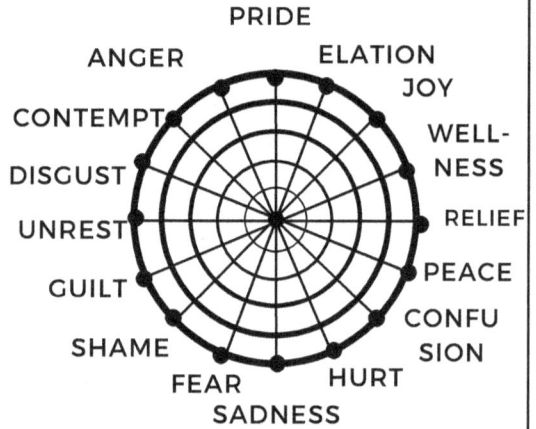

PRIDE

ANGER   ELATION

CONTEMPT   JOY

DISGUST   WELL-NESS

UNREST   RELIEF

GUILT   PEACE

SHAME   CONFU SION

FEAR   HURT

SADNESS

SIDE EFFECTS

_____
_____
_____
_____
_____

Things to celebrate......

_____
_____
_____
_____
_____

NEXT APPOINTMENT DATE & TIME

Check in

Chemo APPOINTMENT DATE _____

HOW AM I FEELING TODAY?

☐ ☐ ☐ ☐ ☐ ☐ ☐ ☐ ☐ ☐

NOT GREAT   INCREDIBLE

Chemotherapy
Center name &
info

SYMPTOMS

_____
_____
_____
_____
_____

DOS

_____
_____
_____
_____
_____
_____

DON'TS

_____
_____
_____
_____

EMOTIONAL WHEEL

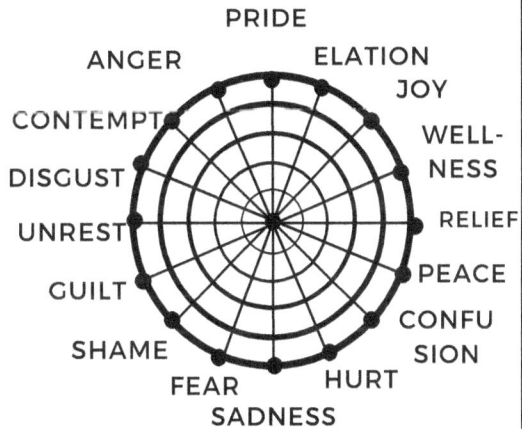

PRIDE
ANGER   ELATION
                    JOY
CONTEMPT
                 WELL-
                 NESS
DISGUST
                  RELIEF
UNREST
               PEACE
GUILT
             CONFU
             SION
SHAME
FEAR   HURT
SADNESS

SIDE EFFECTS

_____
_____
_____
_____
_____

Things to celebrate......

_____
_____
_____
_____
_____

NEXT APPOINTMENT DATE & TIME

Check in

Chemo APPOINTMENT   DATE _____

HOW AM I FEELING TODAY?

☐ ☐ ☐ ☐ ☐ ☐ ☐ ☐ ☐ ☐

NOT GREAT   INCREDIBLE

*chemotherapy
Center name &
info*

DOS

_____

_____

_____

_____

_____

DON'TS

_____

_____

_____

SIDE EFFECTS

_____

_____

_____

_____

_____

SYMPTOMS

_____

_____

_____

_____

_____

EMOTIONAL WHEEL

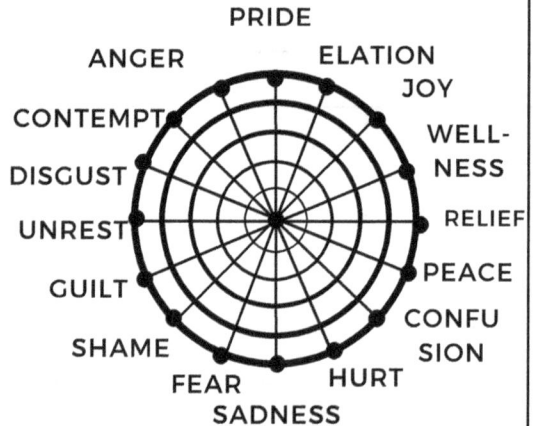

PRIDE
ANGER   ELATION
                    JOY
CONTEMPT
                    WELL-
                    NESS
DISGUST
                    RELIEF
UNREST
                    PEACE
GUILT
                    CONFU
                    SION
SHAME
        FEAR   HURT
        SADNESS

Things to celebrate......

_____

_____

_____

_____

NEXT APPOINTMENT DATE & TIME

Check in

Chemo APPOINTMENT   DATE _____

HOW AM I FEELING TODAY?

☐ ☐ ☐ ☐ ☐ ☐ ☐ ☐ ☐ ☐

NOT GREAT   INCREDIBLE

Chemotherapy Center name & info

SYMPTOMS

_____

_____

_____

_____

_____

DOS

_____

_____

_____

_____

_____

DON'TS

_____

_____

_____

_____

EMOTIONAL WHEEL

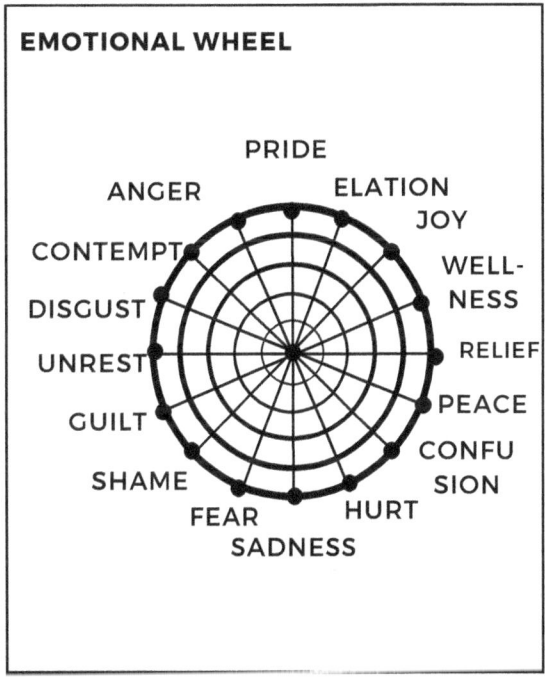

SIDE EFFECTS

_____

_____

_____

_____

_____

Things to celebrate......

_____

_____

_____

_____

_____

NEXT APPOINTMENT DATE & TIME

Check in

Chemo APPOINTMENT DATE _____

HOW AM I FEELING TODAY?

☐ ☐ ☐ ☐ ☐ ☐ ☐ ☐ ☐ ☐

NOT GREAT   INCREDIBLE

chemotherapy Center name & info

DOS

_____

_____

_____

_____

_____

DON'TS

_____

_____

_____

_____

SIDE EFFECTS

_____

_____

_____

_____

_____

SYMPTOMS

_____

_____

_____

_____

_____

EMOTIONAL WHEEL

PRIDE
ANGER   ELATION
                    JOY
CONTEMPT
                WELL-
DISGUST   NESS
                RELIEF
UNREST
                PEACE
GUILT
            CONFU
SHAME   SION
    FEAR   HURT
    SADNESS

Things to celebrate......

_____

_____

_____

_____

NEXT APPOINTMENT DATE & TIME

Check in

Chemo APPOINTMENT   DATE _____

HOW AM I FEELING TODAY?

☐ ☐ ☐ ☐ ☐ ☐ ☐ ☐ ☐ ☐

NOT GREAT   INCREDIBLE

Chemotherapy Center name & info

DOS

_____

_____

_____

_____

_____

DON'TS

_____

_____

_____

_____

SYMPTOMS

_____

_____

_____

_____

_____

EMOTIONAL WHEEL

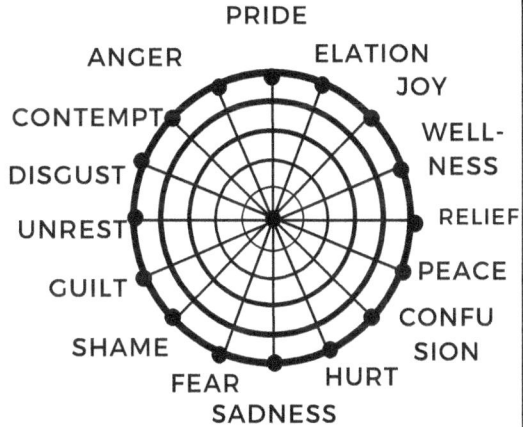

PRIDE
ANGER   ELATION
                    JOY
CONTEMPT   WELL-
                    NESS
DISGUST
                    RELIEF
UNREST
                    PEACE
GUILT
              CONFU
SHAME   SION
      FEAR   HURT
      SADNESS

SIDE EFFECTS

_____

_____

_____

_____

_____

Things to celebrate......

_____

_____

_____

_____

NEXT APPOINTMENT DATE & TIME

Check in

Chemo APPOINTMENT DATE _____

HOW AM I FEELING TODAY?

☐ ☐ ☐ ☐ ☐ ☐ ☐ ☐ ☐ ☐

NOT GREAT   INCREDIBLE

chemotherapy
Center name &
info

DOS

_____
_____
_____
_____
_____

DON'TS

_____
_____
_____

SYMPTOMS

_____
_____
_____
_____
_____

EMOTIONAL WHEEL

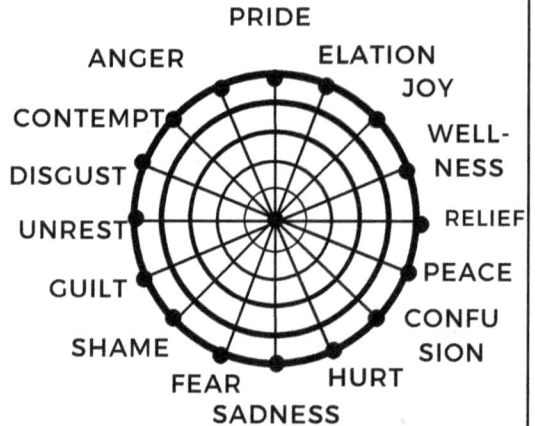

PRIDE

ANGER   ELATION
                   JOY

CONTEMPT   WELL-
                   NESS

DISGUST

UNREST   RELIEF

GUILT   PEACE

SHAME   CONFU
                   SION

FEAR   HURT
SADNESS

SIDE EFFECTS

_____
_____
_____
_____
_____

Things to celebrate......

_____
_____
_____
_____

NEXT APPOINTMENT DATE & TIME

Check in

Chemo   APPOINTMENT   DATE _____

HOW AM I FEELING TODAY?

☐ ☐ ☐ ☐ ☐ ☐ ☐ ☐ ☐ ☐

NOT GREAT   INCREDIBLE

Chemotherapy Center name & info

DOS

_____

_____

_____

_____

_____

DON'TS

_____

_____

_____

SYMPTOMS

_____

_____

_____

_____

_____

EMOTIONAL WHEEL

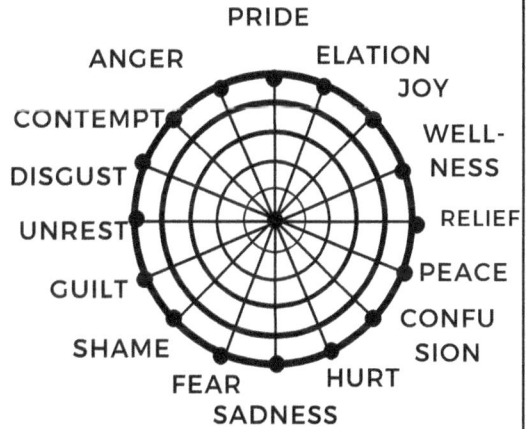

PRIDE
ANGER   ELATION
                  JOY
CONTEMPT
                  WELL-
DISGUST   NESS
UNREST   RELIEF
GUILT   PEACE
                  CONFU
SHAME   SION
   FEAR   HURT
   SADNESS

SIDE EFFECTS

_____

_____

_____

_____

_____

Things to celebrate ......

_____

_____

_____

_____

NEXT APPOINTMENT DATE & TIME

Check in

Chemo APPOINTMENT   DATE _____

HOW AM I FEELING TODAY?

☐ ☐ ☐ ☐ ☐ ☐ ☐ ☐ ☐ ☐

NOT GREAT   INCREDIBLE

chemotherapy
Center name &
info

SYMPTOMS

_____

_____

_____

_____

_____

DOS

_____

_____

_____

_____

_____

DON'TS

_____

_____

_____

EMOTIONAL WHEEL

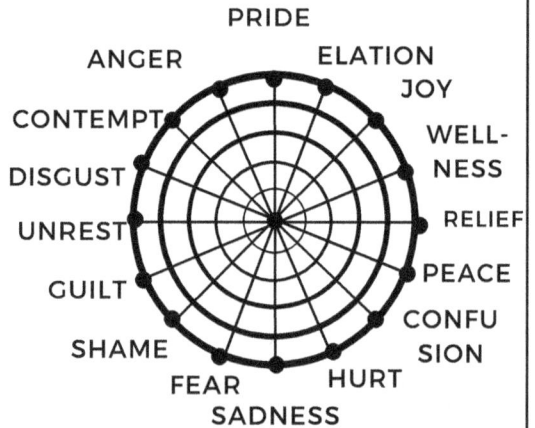

PRIDE

ANGER   ELATION

JOY

CONTEMPT   WELL-
NESS

DISGUST

RELIEF

UNREST

PEACE

GUILT   CONFU
SION

SHAME

FEAR   HURT

SADNESS

SIDE EFFECTS

_____

_____

_____

_____

_____

Things to celebrate......

_____

_____

_____

_____

NEXT APPOINTMENT DATE & TIME

Check in

Chemo APPOINTMENT DATE _____

HOW AM I FEELING TODAY?

☐ ☐ ☐ ☐ ☐ ☐ ☐ ☐ ☐ ☐

NOT GREAT   INCREDIBLE

Chemotherapy Center name & info

SYMPTOMS

_____
_____
_____
_____
_____

DOS

_____
_____
_____
_____
_____

DON'TS

_____
_____
_____

EMOTIONAL WHEEL

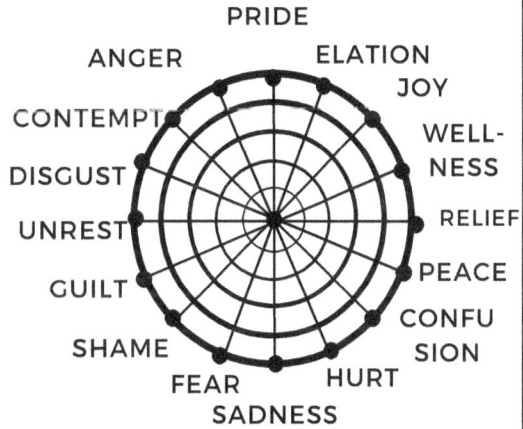

PRIDE
ANGER   ELATION
     JOY
CONTEMPT
    WELL-NESS
DISGUST
UNREST   RELIEF
GUILT   PEACE
CONFU SION
SHAME
FEAR   HURT
SADNESS

SIDE EFFECTS

_____
_____
_____
_____
_____

Things to celebrate......

_____
_____
_____
_____

NEXT APPOINTMENT DATE & TIME

Check in

Chemo APPOINTMENT DATE _____

HOW AM I FEELING TODAY?

☐ ☐ ☐ ☐ ☐ ☐ ☐ ☐ ☐ ☐

NOT GREAT   INCREDIBLE

chemotherapy Center name & info

DOS

_____

_____

_____

_____

_____

_____

DON'TS

_____

_____

_____

SIDE EFFECTS

_____

_____

_____

_____

_____

SYMPTOMS

_____

_____

_____

_____

_____

EMOTIONAL WHEEL

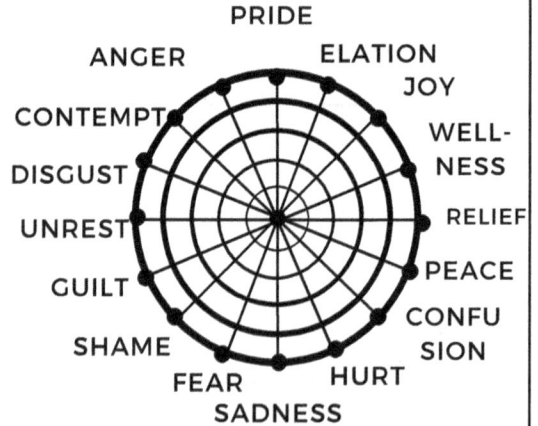

PRIDE
ANGER   ELATION
    JOY
CONTEMPT   WELL-NESS
DISGUST
UNREST   RELIEF
GUILT   PEACE
   CONFUSION
SHAME
FEAR   HURT
SADNESS

Things to celebrate ......

_____

_____

_____

_____

_____

NEXT APPOINTMENT DATE & TIME

Check in

Chemo APPOINTMENT DATE _____

HOW AM I FEELING TODAY?

☐ ☐ ☐ ☐ ☐ ☐ ☐ ☐ ☐ ☐

NOT GREAT   INCREDIBLE

Chemotherapy Center name & info

DOS

_____

_____

_____

_____

_____

_____

DON'TS

_____

_____

_____

SIDE EFFECTS

_____

_____

_____

_____

_____

SYMPTOMS

_____

_____

_____

_____

_____

EMOTIONAL WHEEL

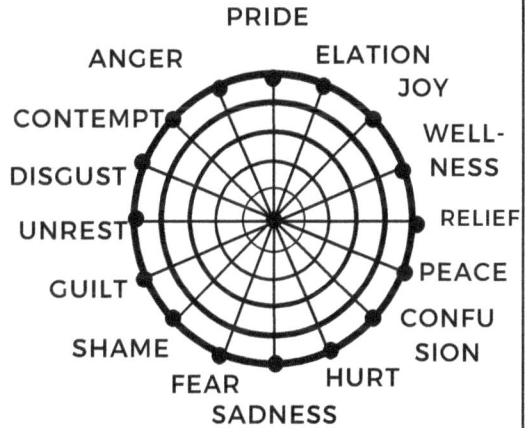

PRIDE
ANGER
ELATION
JOY
CONTEMPT
WELL-NESS
DISGUST
RELIEF
UNREST
PEACE
GUILT
CONFUSION
SHAME
HURT
FEAR
SADNESS

Things to celebrate......

_____

_____

_____

_____

NEXT APPOINTMENT DATE & TIME

Check in

Chemo APPOINTMENT   DATE _____

HOW AM I FEELING TODAY?

☐ ☐ ☐ ☐ ☐ ☐ ☐ ☐ ☐ ☐

NOT GREAT   INCREDIBLE

C

> *chemotherapy
> Center name &
> info*

SYMPTOMS

_____
_____
_____
_____
_____
_____

DOS

_____
_____
_____
_____
_____
_____

DON'TS

_____
_____
_____
_____

EMOTIONAL WHEEL

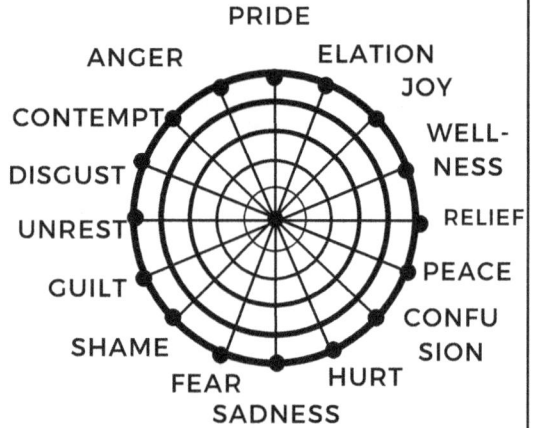

PRIDE
ANGER   ELATION
                      JOY
CONTEMPT
                  WELL-
DISGUST   NESS
UNREST   RELIEF
                  PEACE
GUILT   CONFU
                SION
SHAME   HURT
  FEAR
  SADNESS

SIDE EFFECTS

_____
_____
_____
_____
_____

Things to celebrate ......

_____
_____
_____
_____
_____

NEXT APPOINTMENT DATE & TIME

Check in

Chemo APPOINTMENT   DATE _____

HOW AM I FEELING TODAY?

☐ ☐ ☐ ☐ ☐ ☐ ☐ ☐ ☐ ☐

NOT GREAT   INCREDIBLE

Chemotherapy
Center name &
info

DOS

_____
_____
_____
_____
_____
_____

DON'TS

_____
_____
_____
_____

SYMPTOMS

_____
_____
_____
_____
_____
_____

EMOTIONAL WHEEL

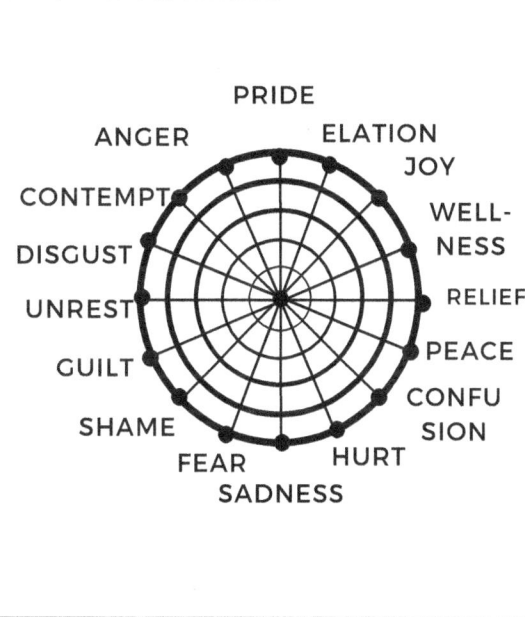

PRIDE
ANGER   ELATION
                 JOY
CONTEMPT
                 WELL-
DISGUST   NESS
UNREST   RELIEF
                 PEACE
GUILT
               CONFU
SHAME   SION
      FEAR   HURT
      SADNESS

SIDE EFFECTS

_____
_____
_____
_____
_____

Things to celebrate......

_____
_____
_____
_____
_____

NEXT APPOINTMENT DATE & TIME

Check in

Chemo APPOINTMENT   DATE _____

HOW AM I FEELING TODAY?

☐ ☐ ☐ ☐ ☐ ☐ ☐ ☐ ☐ ☐

NOT GREAT   INCREDIBLE

*chemotherapy
Center name &
info*

DOS

_____
_____
_____
_____
_____

DON'TS

_____
_____
_____
_____

SIDE EFFECTS

_____
_____
_____
_____
_____

SYMPTOMS

_____
_____
_____
_____
_____

EMOTIONAL WHEEL

PRIDE
ANGER   ELATION   JOY
CONTEMPT   WELL-NESS
DISGUST   RELIEF
UNREST   PEACE
GUILT   CONFUSION
SHAME   HURT
FEAR   SADNESS

Things to celebrate......

_____
_____
_____
_____
_____

NEXT APPOINTMENT DATE & TIME

Check in

Chemo APPOINTMENT DATE _____

HOW AM I FEELING TODAY?

☐ ☐ ☐ ☐ ☐ ☐ ☐ ☐ ☐ ☐

NOT GREAT   INCREDIBLE

Chemotherapy Center name & info

SYMPTOMS

_____
_____
_____
_____
_____

DOS

_____
_____
_____
_____
_____

EMOTIONAL WHEEL

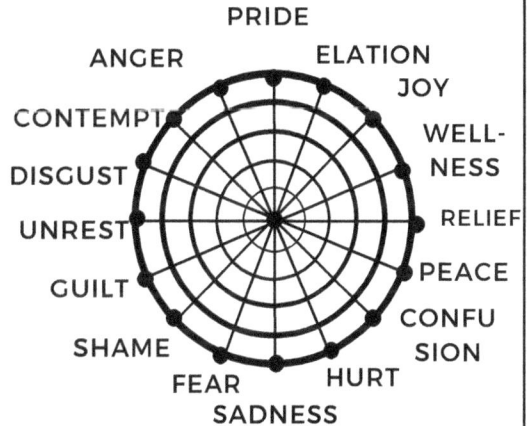

DON'TS

_____
_____
_____
_____

SIDE EFFECTS

_____
_____
_____
_____
_____

Things to celebrate......

_____
_____
_____
_____

NEXT APPOINTMENT DATE & TIME

Check in

Chemo APPOINTMENT DATE _____

HOW AM I FEELING TODAY?

☐ ☐ ☐ ☐ ☐ ☐ ☐ ☐ ☐ ☐

NOT GREAT   INCREDIBLE

*chemotherapy
Center name &
info*

SYMPTOMS

_____
_____
_____
_____
_____

DOS

_____
_____
_____
_____
_____

DON'TS

_____
_____
_____
_____

EMOTIONAL WHEEL

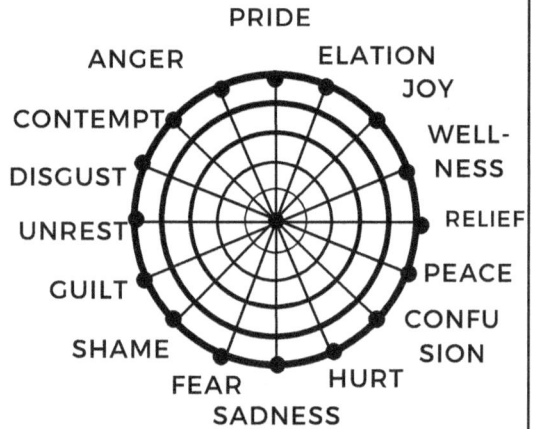

PRIDE
ANGER   ELATION
                    JOY
CONTEMPT   WELL-
                NESS
DISGUST
UNREST   RELIEF
GUILT   PEACE
                CONFU
SHAME   SION
      FEAR   HURT
      SADNESS

SIDE EFFECTS

_____
_____
_____
_____
_____

Things to celebrate.....

_____
_____
_____
_____
_____

NEXT APPOINTMENT DATE & TIME

Check in

Chemo APPOINTMENT   DATE _____

HOW AM I FEELING TODAY?

☐ ☐ ☐ ☐ ☐ ☐ ☐ ☐ ☐ ☐

NOT GREAT   INCREDIBLE

Chemotherapy
Center name &
info

SYMPTOMS

_____
_____
_____
_____
_____
_____

DOS

_____
_____
_____
_____
_____

DON'TS

_____
_____
_____
_____

EMOTIONAL WHEEL

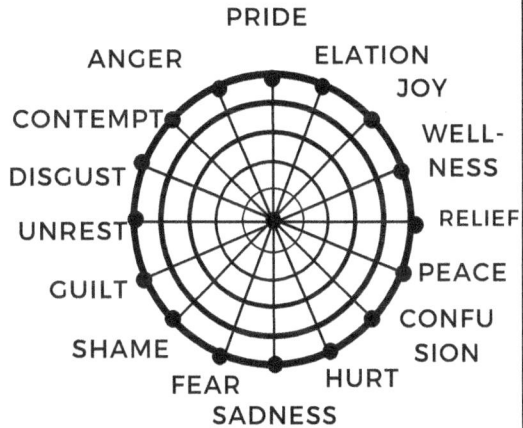

PRIDE
ANGER   ELATION
JOY
CONTEMPT   WELL-NESS
DISGUST
UNREST   RELIEF
GUILT   PEACE
CONFUSION
SHAME
FEAR   HURT
SADNESS

SIDE EFFECTS

_____
_____
_____
_____
_____

Things to celebrate......

_____
_____
_____
_____
_____

NEXT APPOINTMENT DATE & TIME

Check in

Chemo APPOINTMENT   DATE _____

HOW AM I FEELING TODAY?

☐ ☐ ☐ ☐ ☐ ☐ ☐ ☐ ☐ ☐

NOT GREAT   INCREDIBLE

C

chemotherapy Center name & info

SYMPTOMS

_____

_____

_____

_____

_____

DOS

_____

_____

_____

_____

_____

DON'TS

_____

_____

_____

EMOTIONAL WHEEL

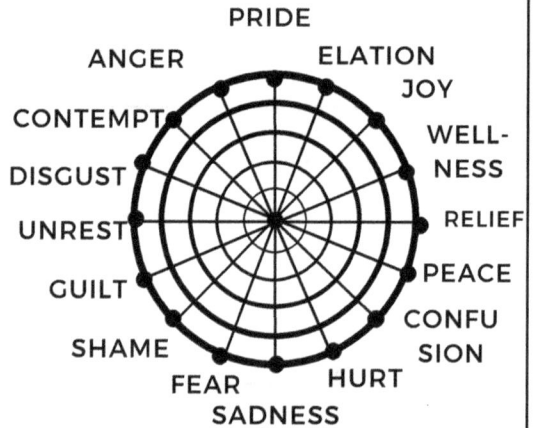

PRIDE

ANGER   ELATION

JOY

CONTEMPT   WELL-NESS

DISGUST   RELIEF

UNREST   PEACE

GUILT   CONFUSION

SHAME   HURT

FEAR   SADNESS

SIDE EFFECTS

_____

_____

_____

_____

_____

Things to celebrate......

_____

_____

_____

_____

NEXT APPOINTMENT DATE & TIME

Check in

Chemo APPOINTMENT   DATE _____

HOW AM I FEELING TODAY?

☐ ☐ ☐ ☐ ☐ ☐ ☐ ☐ ☐ ☐

NOT GREAT   INCREDIBLE

Chemotherapy Center name & info

SYMPTOMS

_____
_____
_____
_____
_____

DOS

_____
_____
_____
_____
_____
_____

DON'TS

_____
_____
_____

EMOTIONAL WHEEL

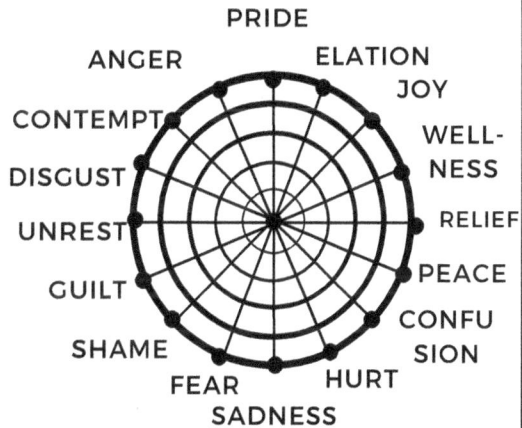

PRIDE
ANGER   ELATION
CONTEMPT   JOY
DISGUST   WELL-NESS
UNREST   RELIEF
GUILT   PEACE
SHAME   CONFUSION
FEAR   HURT
SADNESS

SIDE EFFECTS

_____
_____
_____
_____
_____

Things to celebrate......

_____
_____
_____
_____
_____

NEXT APPOINTMENT DATE & TIME

Check in

Chemo APPOINTMENT   DATE _____

HOW AM I FEELING TODAY?

☐ ☐ ☐ ☐ ☐ ☐ ☐ ☐ ☐ ☐

NOT GREAT   INCREDIBLE

C

> *chemotherapy Center name & info*

SYMPTOMS

_____

_____

_____

_____

_____

DOS

_____

_____

_____

_____

_____

_____

DON'TS

_____

_____

_____

EMOTIONAL WHEEL

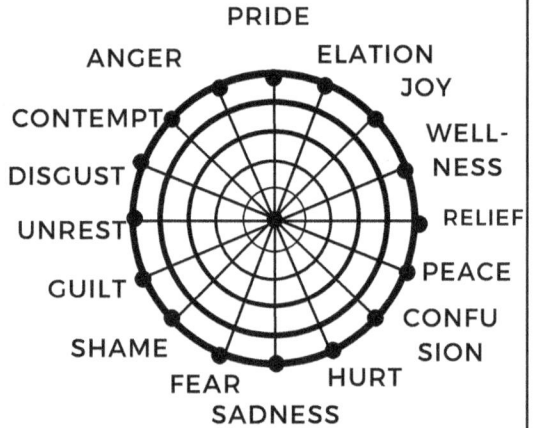

PRIDE
ANGER   ELATION
          JOY
CONTEMPT
          WELL-
DISGUST   NESS
          RELIEF
UNREST
          PEACE
GUILT   CONFU
          SION
SHAME
      HURT
FEAR
SADNESS

SIDE EFFECTS

_____

_____

_____

_____

_____

Things to celebrate......

_____

_____

_____

_____

_____

NEXT APPOINTMENT DATE & TIME

Check in

Chemo APPOINTMENT   DATE _____

HOW AM I FEELING TODAY?

☐ ☐ ☐ ☐ ☐ ☐ ☐ ☐ ☐ ☐

NOT GREAT   INCREDIBLE

Chemotherapy Center name & info

DOS

_____

_____

_____

_____

_____

DON'TS

_____

_____

_____

SIDE EFFECTS

_____

_____

_____

_____

_____

SYMPTOMS

_____

_____

_____

_____

_____

EMOTIONAL WHEEL

PRIDE
ANGER   ELATION
                    JOY
CONTEMPT
                    WELL-
DISGUST   NESS
UNREST   RELIEF
GUILT   PEACE
SHAME   CONFU
                SION
FEAR   HURT
SADNESS

Things to celebrate......

_____

_____

_____

_____

NEXT APPOINTMENT DATE & TIME

Check in

Chemo APPOINTMENT   DATE _____

HOW AM I FEELING TODAY?

☐ ☐ ☐ ☐ ☐ ☐ ☐ ☐ ☐ ☐

NOT GREAT   INCREDIBLE

C

chemotherapy Center name & info

SYMPTOMS

_____
_____
_____
_____
_____

DOS

_____
_____
_____
_____
_____

DON'TS

_____
_____
_____
_____

EMOTIONAL WHEEL

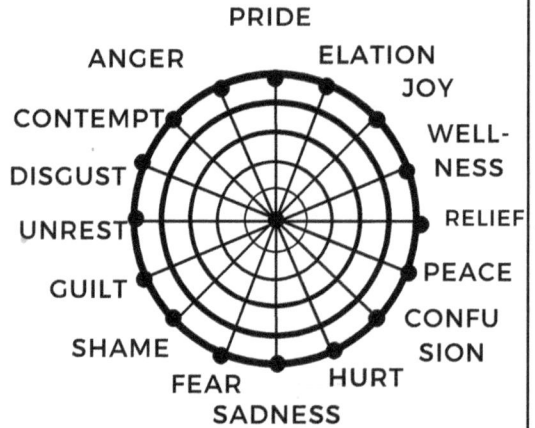

PRIDE
ANGER   ELATION
                JOY
CONTEMPT   WELL-
                   NESS
DISGUST
UNREST   RELIEF
GUILT   PEACE
                  CONFU
SHAME   SION
     FEAR   HURT
     SADNESS

SIDE EFFECTS

_____
_____
_____
_____
_____

Things to celebrate......

_____
_____
_____
_____
_____

NEXT APPOINTMENT DATE & TIME

Check in

Chemo APPOINTMENT   DATE _____

HOW AM I FEELING TODAY?

☐ ☐ ☐ ☐ ☐ ☐ ☐ ☐ ☐ ☐

NOT GREAT   INCREDIBLE

Chemotherapy Center name & info

SYMPTOMS

_____
_____
_____
_____
_____

DOS

_____
_____
_____
_____
_____

DON'TS

_____
_____
_____
_____

EMOTIONAL WHEEL

PRIDE
ANGER   ELATION
                 JOY
CONTEMPT
               WELL-
DISGUST   NESS

UNREST   RELIEF

GUILT   PEACE

SHAME   CONFU
              SION
   FEAR   HURT
    SADNESS

SIDE EFFECTS

_____
_____
_____
_____
_____

Things to celebrate......

_____
_____
_____
_____

NEXT APPOINTMENT DATE & TIME

Check in

Chemo APPOINTMENT DATE _____

HOW AM I FEELING TODAY?

☐ ☐ ☐ ☐ ☐ ☐ ☐ ☐ ☐ ☐
NOT GREAT   INCREDIBLE

C

> *chemotherapy
> Center name &
> info*

SYMPTOMS

_____
_____
_____
_____
_____

DOS

_____
_____
_____
_____
_____

EMOTIONAL WHEEL

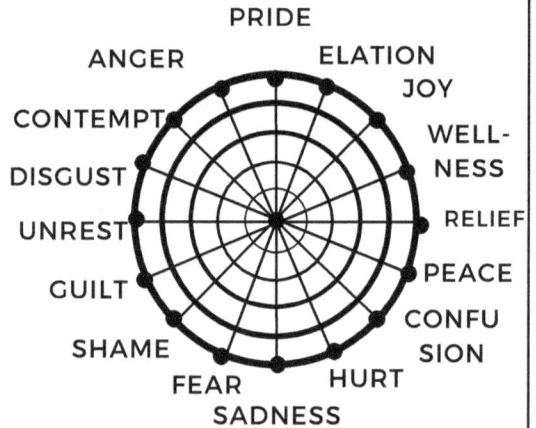

PRIDE
ANGER   ELATION
                    JOY
CONTEMPT
                    WELL-
                    NESS
DISGUST
                    RELIEF
UNREST
                    PEACE
GUILT
                    CONFU
                    SION
SHAME
        FEAR   HURT
        SADNESS

DON'TS

_____
_____
_____

SIDE EFFECTS

_____
_____
_____
_____
_____

Things to celebrate......

_____
_____
_____
_____
_____

NEXT APPOINTMENT DATE & TIME

Check in

Chemo APPOINTMENT   DATE _____

HOW AM I FEELING TODAY?

☐ ☐ ☐ ☐ ☐ ☐ ☐ ☐ ☐ ☐

NOT GREAT   INCREDIBLE

Chemotherapy Center name & info

DOS

_____

_____

_____

_____

_____

DON'TS

_____

_____

_____

_____

SIDE EFFECTS

_____

_____

_____

_____

_____

SYMPTOMS

_____

_____

_____

_____

_____

EMOTIONAL WHEEL

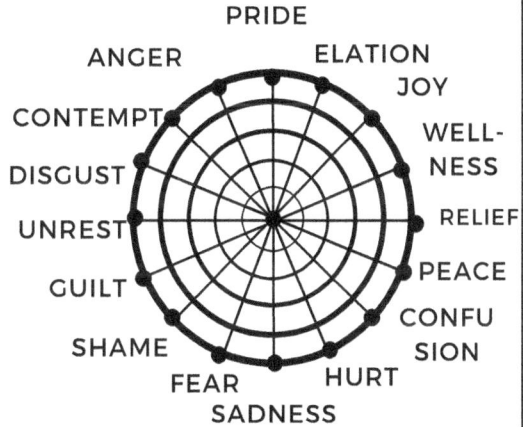

PRIDE · ANGER · ELATION · JOY · CONTEMPT · WELLNESS · DISGUST · RELIEF · UNREST · PEACE · GUILT · CONFUSION · SHAME · HURT · FEAR · SADNESS

Things to celebrate......

_____

_____

_____

_____

_____

NEXT APPOINTMENT DATE & TIME

Check in

Surgery APPOINTMENT DATE _____

HOW AM I FEELING TODAY?

☐ ☐ ☐ ☐ ☐ ☐ ☐ ☐ ☐ ☐

NOT GREAT   INCREDIBLE

Surgery Center
name & info

DOS

_____

_____

_____

_____

_____

DON'TS

_____

_____

_____

_____

SYMPTOMS

_____

_____

_____

_____

_____

EMOTIONAL WHEEL

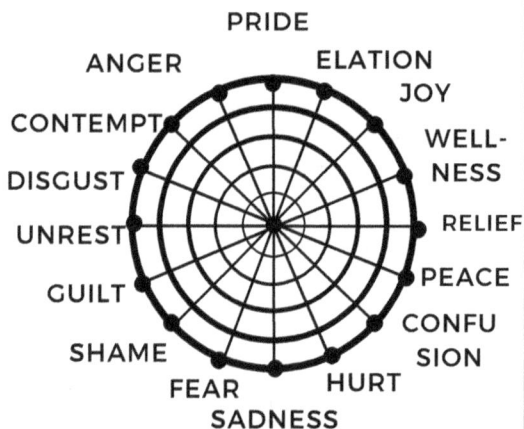

PRIDE
ANGER   ELATION
                    JOY
CONTEMPT
                    WELL-
DISGUST   NESS
UNREST   RELIEF
                    PEACE
GUILT   CONFU
                    SION
SHAME
         FEAR   HURT
         SADNESS

SIDE EFFECTS

_____

_____

_____

_____

_____

Things to celebrate......

_____

_____

_____

_____

_____

NEXT APPOINTMENT DATE & TIME

Check in

Surgery APPOINTMENT DATE _____

HOW AM I FEELING TODAY?

☐ ☐ ☐ ☐ ☐ ☐ ☐ ☐ ☐ ☐

NOT GREAT   INCREDIBLE

Surgery Center name & info

DOS

_____
_____
_____
_____
_____

DON'TS

_____
_____
_____

SYMPTOMS

_____
_____
_____
_____
_____

EMOTIONAL WHEEL

PRIDE
ANGER   ELATION
                    JOY
CONTEMPT   WELL-
                    NESS
DISGUST
UNREST   RELIEF
GUILT   PEACE
                CONFU
SHAME   SION
     FEAR   HURT
     SADNESS

SIDE EFFECTS

_____
_____
_____
_____
_____

Things to celebrate ......

_____
_____
_____
_____

NEXT APPOINTMENT DATE & TIME

Check in

Surgery APPOINTMENT   DATE _____

HOW AM I FEELING TODAY?

☐ ☐ ☐ ☐ ☐ ☐ ☐ ☐ ☐ ☐

NOT GREAT   INCREDIBLE

*Surgery Center
name & info*

DOS

_____
_____
_____
_____
_____
_____

DON'TS

_____
_____
_____
_____

SIDE EFFECTS

_____
_____
_____
_____
_____

SYMPTOMS

_____
_____
_____
_____
_____

EMOTIONAL WHEEL

PRIDE
ANGER   ELATION
                JOY
CONTEMPT
                WELL-
DISGUST   NESS
                RELIEF
UNREST
                PEACE
GUILT   CONFU
                SION
SHAME   HURT
    FEAR
    SADNESS

Things to celebrate......

_____
_____
_____
_____
_____

NEXT APPOINTMENT DATE & TIME

Check in

Surgery APPOINTMENT   DATE _____

HOW AM I FEELING TODAY?

☐ ☐ ☐ ☐ ☐ ☐ ☐ ☐ ☐ ☐

NOT GREAT   INCREDIBLE

*Surgery Center
name & info*

SYMPTOMS

_____
_____
_____
_____
_____

DOS

_____
_____
_____
_____
_____

DON'TS

_____
_____
_____

EMOTIONAL WHEEL

PRIDE
ANGER   ELATION
                    JOY
CONTEMPT   WELL-
                 NESS
DISGUST
                 RELIEF
UNREST
                 PEACE
GUILT
                 CONFU
SHAME   SION
        FEAR   HURT
        SADNESS

SIDE EFFECTS

_____
_____
_____
_____
_____

Things to celebrate......

_____
_____
_____
_____
_____

NEXT APPOINTMENT DATE & TIME

Check in

Surgery APPOINTMENT   DATE _____

HOW AM I FEELING TODAY?

☐ ☐ ☐ ☐ ☐ ☐ ☐ ☐ ☐ ☐

NOT GREAT   INCREDIBLE

Surgery Center
name & info

DOS

_____
_____
_____
_____
_____

DON'TS

_____
_____
_____
_____

SIDE EFFECTS

_____
_____
_____
_____
_____

SYMPTOMS

_____
_____
_____
_____
_____

EMOTIONAL WHEEL

PRIDE
ELATION
ANGER
JOY
CONTEMPT
WELL-NESS
DISGUST
UNREST
RELIEF
GUILT
PEACE
CONFU SION
SHAME
HURT
FEAR
SADNESS

Things to celebrate......

_____
_____
_____
_____

NEXT APPOINTMENT DATE & TIME

Check in

Surgery APPOINTMENT

DATE _____

HOW AM I FEELING TODAY?

☐ ☐ ☐ ☐ ☐ ☐ ☐ ☐ ☐ ☐

NOT GREAT   INCREDIBLE

Surgery Center
name & info

DOS

_____
_____
_____
_____
_____

DON'TS

_____
_____
_____
_____

SYMPTOMS

_____
_____
_____
_____
_____

EMOTIONAL WHEEL

PRIDE
ANGER   ELATION
                JOY
CONTEMPT   WELL-
               NESS
DISGUST
               RELIEF
UNREST
               PEACE
GUILT   CONFU
               SION
SHAME
      FEAR   HURT
      SADNESS

SIDE EFFECTS

_____
_____
_____
_____
_____

Things to celebrate......

_____
_____
_____
_____

NEXT APPOINTMENT DATE & TIME

Daily routine

____ / ____ / ____

M T W T F S S

OUTSIDE TIME

TIME	LENGTH

BATHROOM TIME

	wet	b.m.
	wet	b.m.
	wet	b.m.
	wet	b.m.

SLEEP TIME

TIME	LENGTH

Snacks

MY DAY WAS

○ Good   ○ Fair   ○ Poor

Meals

Morning	○ Good	○ Fair	○ Poor
Evening	○ Good	○ Fair	○ Poor

DAILY GOALS

ACTIVITY	LENGTH	MEDICINE	TIME	DOSAGE

SEXUAL HEALTH

SYMPTOMS	RATE				
	Very Poor	Poor	Fair	Good	Excellent
	○	○	○	○	○
	○	○	○	○	○
	○	○	○	○	○
	○	○	○	○	○
	○	○	○	○	○

NOTES

Daily routine

____ / ____ / ____

M	T	W	T	F	S	S
•	•	•	•	•	•	•

OUTSIDE TIME

TIME	LENGTH

BATHROOM TIME

	wet	b.m.
	wet	b.m.
	wet	b.m.
	wet	b.m.

SLEEP TIME

TIME	LENGTH

Snacks

MY DAY WAS

○ **Good**   ○ **Fair**   ○ **Poor**

Meals

Morning	○ Good	○ Fair	○ Poor
Evening	○ Good	○ Fair	○ Poor

DAILY GOALS

ACTIVITY	LENGTH	MEDICINE	TIME	DOSAGE

SEXUAL HEALTH

SYMPTOMS	RATE				
	Very Poor	Poor	Fair	Good	Excellent
	○	○	○	○	○
	○	○	○	○	○
	○	○	○	○	○
	○	○	○	○	○
	○	○	○	○	○

NOTES

241

Daily routine

____ / ____ / ____

M	T	W	T	F	S	S
●	●	●	●	●	●	●

OUTSIDE TIME

TIME	LENGTH

BATHROOM TIME

		wet	b.m.
		wet	b.m.
		wet	b.m.
		wet	b.m.

SLEEP TIME

TIME	LENGTH

Snacks

MY DAY WAS

○ **Good**   ○ **Fair**   ○ **Poor**

Meals

Morning	○ Good	○ Fair	○ Poor
Evening	○ Good	○ Fair	○ Poor

DAILY GOALS

ACTIVITY	LENGTH	MEDICINE	TIME	DOSAGE

SEXUAL HEALTH

SYMPTOMS	RATE				
	Very Poor	Poor	Fair	Good	Excellent
	○	○	○	○	○
	○	○	○	○	○
	○	○	○	○	○
	○	○	○	○	○
	○	○	○	○	○

NOTES

Daily routine

____ / ____ / ____

| M | T | W | T | F | S | S |

OUTSIDE TIME

TIME	LENGTH

BATHROOM TIME

		wet	b.m.
		wet	b.m.
		wet	b.m.
		wet	b.m.

SLEEP TIME

TIME	LENGTH

Snacks

MY DAY WAS

○ **Good**   ○ **Fair**   ○ **Poor**

Meals

Morning	○ **Good**	○ **Fair**	○ **Poor**
Evening	○ **Good**	○ **Fair**	○ **Poor**

DAILY GOALS

ACTIVITY	LENGTH	MEDICINE	TIME	DOSAGE

SEXUAL HEALTH

SYMPTOMS	RATE				
	Very Poor	Poor	Fair	Good	Excellent
	○	○	○	○	○
	○	○	○	○	○
	○	○	○	○	○
	○	○	○	○	○
	○	○	○	○	○

NOTES

Daily routine

____ / ____ / ____

| M | T | W | T | F | S | S |

OUTSIDE TIME

TIME	LENGTH

BATHROOM TIME

	wet	b.m.
	wet	b.m.
	wet	b.m.
	wet	b.m.

SLEEP TIME

TIME	LENGTH

Snacks

MY DAY WAS

○ **Good**   ○ **Fair**   ○ **Poor**

Meals

| **Morning** | ○ **Good** | ○ **Fair** | ○ **Poor** |
| **Evening** | ○ **Good** | ○ **Fair** | ○ **Poor** |

DAILY GOALS

ACTIVITY	LENGTH	MEDICINE	TIME	DOSAGE

SEXUAL HEALTH

SYMPTOMS	RATE				
	Very Poor	Poor	Fair	Good	Excellent
	○	○	○	○	○
	○	○	○	○	○
	○	○	○	○	○
	○	○	○	○	○
	○	○	○	○	○

NOTES

Daily routine

____ / ____ / ____

M	T	W	T	F	S	S
•	•	•	•	•	•	•

OUTSIDE TIME

TIME	LENGTH

BATHROOM TIME

	wet	b.m.
	wet	b.m.
	wet	b.m.
	wet	b.m.

SLEEP TIME

TIME	LENGTH

Snacks

MY DAY WAS

○ **Good**   ○ **Fair**   ○ **Poor**

Meals

Morning	○ **Good**	○ **Fair**	○ **Poor**
Evening	○ **Good**	○ **Fair**	○ **Poor**

DAILY GOALS

ACTIVITY	LENGTH	MEDICINE	TIME	DOSAGE

SEXUAL HEALTH

SYMPTOMS	RATE				
	Very Poor	Poor	Fair	Good	Excellent
	○	○	○	○	○
	○	○	○	○	○
	○	○	○	○	○
	○	○	○	○	○
	○	○	○	○	○

NOTES

245

Daily routine

____ / ____ / ____

M	T	W	T	F	S	S
●	●	●	●	●	●	●

OUTSIDE TIME

TIME	LENGTH

BATHROOM TIME

	wet	b.m.
	wet	b.m.
	wet	b.m.
	wet	b.m.

SLEEP TIME

TIME	LENGTH

Snacks

MY DAY WAS

○ Good   ○ Fair   ○ Poor

Meals

Morning	○ Good	○ Fair	○ Poor
Evening	○ Good	○ Fair	○ Poor

DAILY GOALS

ACTIVITY	LENGTH	MEDICINE	TIME	DOSAGE

SEXUAL HEALTH

SYMPTOMS	RATE				
	Very Poor	Poor	Fair	Good	Excellent
	○	○	○	○	○
	○	○	○	○	○
	○	○	○	○	○
	○	○	○	○	○
	○	○	○	○	○

NOTES

Daily routine

____ / ____ / ____

M	T	W	T	F	S	S
●	●	●	●	●	●	●

OUTSIDE TIME

TIME	LENGTH

BATHROOM TIME

	wet	b.m.
	wet	b.m.
	wet	b.m.
	wet	b.m.

SLEEP TIME

TIME	LENGTH

Snacks

MY DAY WAS

○ **Good**   ○ **Fair**   ○ **Poor**

Meals

Morning	○ **Good**	○ **Fair**	○ **Poor**
Evening	○ **Good**	○ **Fair**	○ **Poor**

DAILY GOALS

ACTIVITY	LENGTH	MEDICINE	TIME	DOSAGE

SEXUAL HEALTH

SYMPTOMS	RATE				
	Very Poor	Poor	Fair	Good	Excellent
	○	○	○	○	○
	○	○	○	○	○
	○	○	○	○	○
	○	○	○	○	○
	○	○	○	○	○

NOTES

Daily routine

____ / ____ / ____

M T W T F S S
● ● ● ● ● ● ●

OUTSIDE TIME

TIME	LENGTH

BATHROOM TIME

	wet	b.m.
	wet	b.m.
	wet	b.m.
	wet	b.m.

SLEEP TIME

TIME	LENGTH

Snacks

MY DAY WAS

○ Good   ○ Fair   ○ Poor

Meals

Morning	○ Good	○ Fair	○ Poor
Evening	○ Good	○ Fair	○ Poor

DAILY GOALS

ACTIVITY	LENGTH	MEDICINE	TIME	DOSAGE

SEXUAL HEALTH

SYMPTOMS	RATE				
	Very Poor	Poor	Fair	Good	Excellent
	○	○	○	○	○
	○	○	○	○	○
	○	○	○	○	○
	○	○	○	○	○
	○	○	○	○	○

NOTES

Daily routine

____ / ____ / ____

M	T	W	T	F	S	S
●	●	●	●	●	●	●

OUTSIDE TIME

TIME	LENGTH

BATHROOM TIME

	wet	b.m.
	wet	b.m.
	wet	b.m.
	wet	b.m.

SLEEP TIME

TIME	LENGTH

Snacks

MY DAY WAS

○ **Good**   ○ **Fair**   ○ **Poor**

Meals

Morning	○ Good	○ Fair	○ Poor
Evening	○ Good	○ Fair	○ Poor

DAILY GOALS

ACTIVITY	LENGTH	MEDICINE	TIME	DOSAGE

SEXUAL HEALTH

SYMPTOMS	RATE				
	Very Poor	Poor	Fair	Good	Excellent
	○	○	○	○	○
	○	○	○	○	○
	○	○	○	○	○
	○	○	○	○	○
	○	○	○	○	○

NOTES

249

Daily routine

____ / ____ / ____

M	T	W	T	F	S	S
●	●	●	●	●	●	●

OUTSIDE TIME

TIME	LENGTH

BATHROOM TIME

	wet	b.m.
	wet	b.m.
	wet	b.m.
	wet	b.m.

SLEEP TIME

TIME	LENGTH

Snacks

MY DAY WAS

○ **Good**   ○ **Fair**   ○ **Poor**

Meals

Morning	○ **Good**	○ **Fair**	○ **Poor**
Evening	○ **Good**	○ **Fair**	○ **Poor**

DAILY GOALS

ACTIVITY	LENGTH	MEDICINE	TIME	DOSAGE

SEXUAL HEALTH

SYMPTOMS	RATE				
	Very Poor	Poor	Fair	Good	Excellent
	○	○	○	○	○
	○	○	○	○	○
	○	○	○	○	○
	○	○	○	○	○
	○	○	○	○	○

NOTES

Daily routine

_____ / _____ / _____

M	T	W	T	F	S	S
●	●	●	●	●	●	●

OUTSIDE TIME

TIME	LENGTH

BATHROOM TIME

		wet	b.m.
		wet	b.m.
		wet	b.m.
		wet	b.m.

SLEEP TIME

TIME	LENGTH

Snacks

MY DAY WAS

○ **Good**   ○ **Fair**   ○ **Poor**

Meals

Morning	○ **Good**	○ **Fair**	○ **Poor**
Evening	○ **Good**	○ **Fair**	○ **Poor**

DAILY GOALS

ACTIVITY	LENGTH	MEDICINE	TIME	DOSAGE

SEXUAL HEALTH

SYMPTOMS	RATE				
	Very Poor	Poor	Fair	Good	Excellent
	○	○	○	○	○
	○	○	○	○	○
	○	○	○	○	○
	○	○	○	○	○
	○	○	○	○	○

NOTES

Daily routine

____ / ___ / ___

M   T   W   T   F   S   S

OUTSIDE TIME

TIME	LENGTH

BATHROOM TIME

	wet	b.m.
	wet	b.m.
	wet	b.m.
	wet	b.m.

SLEEP TIME

TIME	LENGTH

Snacks

MY DAY WAS

○ **Good**   ○ **Fair**   ○ **Poor**

Meals

Morning	○ Good	○ Fair	○ Poor
Evening	○ Good	○ Fair	○ Poor

DAILY GOALS

ACTIVITY	LENGTH	MEDICINE	TIME	DOSAGE

SEXUAL HEALTH

SYMPTOMS	RATE				
	Very Poor	Poor	Fair	Good	Excellent
	○	○	○	○	○
	○	○	○	○	○
	○	○	○	○	○
	○	○	○	○	○
	○	○	○	○	○

NOTES

Daily routine

____ / ____ / ____

M	T	W	T	F	S	S
•	•	•	•	•	•	•

OUTSIDE TIME

TIME	LENGTH

BATHROOM TIME

	wet	b.m.
	wet	b.m.
	wet	b.m.
	wet	b.m.

SLEEP TIME

TIME	LENGTH

Snacks

MY DAY WAS

○ **Good**   ○ **Fair**   ○ **Poor**

Meals

Morning	○ **Good**	○ **Fair**	○ **Poor**
Evening	○ **Good**	○ **Fair**	○ **Poor**

DAILY GOALS

ACTIVITY	LENGTH	MEDICINE	TIME	DOSAGE

SEXUAL HEALTH

SYMPTOMS	RATE				
	Very Poor	Poor	Fair	Good	Excellent
	○	○	○	○	○
	○	○	○	○	○
	○	○	○	○	○
	○	○	○	○	○
	○	○	○	○	○

NOTES

Daily routine

___ / ___ / ___

M	T	W	T	F	S	S
●	●	●	●	●	●	●

OUTSIDE TIME

TIME	LENGTH

BATHROOM TIME

		wet	b.m.
		wet	b.m.
		wet	b.m.
		wet	b.m.

SLEEP TIME

TIME	LENGTH

Snacks

MY DAY WAS

○ **Good**   ○ **Fair**   ○ **Poor**

Meals

Morning	○ **Good**	○ **Fair**	○ **Poor**
Evening	○ **Good**	○ **Fair**	○ **Poor**

DAILY GOALS

ACTIVITY	LENGTH	MEDICINE	TIME	DOSAGE

SEXUAL HEALTH

SYMPTOMS	RATE				
	Very Poor	Poor	Fair	Good	Excellent
	○	○	○	○	○
	○	○	○	○	○
	○	○	○	○	○
	○	○	○	○	○
	○	○	○	○	○

NOTES

Daily routine

____ / ____ / ____

M	T	W	T	F	S	S
●	●	●	●	●	●	●

OUTSIDE TIME

TIME	LENGTH

BATHROOM TIME

	wet	b.m.
	wet	b.m.
	wet	b.m.
	wet	b.m.

SLEEP TIME

TIME	LENGTH

Snacks

MY DAY WAS

○ **Good**   ○ **Fair**   ○ **Poor**

Meals

Morning	○ Good	○ Fair	○ Poor
Evening	○ Good	○ Fair	○ Poor

DAILY GOALS

ACTIVITY	LENGTH	MEDICINE	TIME	DOSAGE

SEXUAL HEALTH

SYMPTOMS	RATE				
	Very Poor	Poor	Fair	Good	Excellent
	○	○	○	○	○
	○	○	○	○	○
	○	○	○	○	○
	○	○	○	○	○
	○	○	○	○	○

NOTES

Daily routine

____ / ____ / ____

| M | T | W | T | F | S | S |

OUTSIDE TIME

TIME	LENGTH

BATHROOM TIME

	wet	b.m.
	wet	b.m.
	wet	b.m.
	wet	b.m.

SLEEP TIME

TIME	LENGTH

Snacks

MY DAY WAS

○ Good   ○ Fair   ○ Poor

Meals

Morning	○ Good	○ Fair	○ Poor
Evening	○ Good	○ Fair	○ Poor

DAILY GOALS

ACTIVITY	LENGTH	MEDICINE	TIME	DOSAGE

SEXUAL HEALTH

SYMPTOMS	RATE				
	Very Poor	Poor	Fair	Good	Excellent
	○	○	○	○	○
	○	○	○	○	○
	○	○	○	○	○
	○	○	○	○	○
	○	○	○	○	○

NOTES

Daily routine

____ / ____ / ____

M   T   W   T   F   S   S
●   ●   ●   ●   ●   ●   ●

OUTSIDE TIME

TIME	LENGTH

BATHROOM TIME

	wet	b.m.
	wet	b.m.
	wet	b.m.
	wet	b.m.

SLEEP TIME

TIME	LENGTH

Snacks

MY DAY WAS

○ Good   ○ Fair   ○ Poor

Meals

Morning	○ Good	○ Fair	○ Poor
Evening	○ Good	○ Fair	○ Poor

DAILY GOALS

ACTIVITY	LENGTH	MEDICINE	TIME	DOSAGE

SEXUAL HEALTH

SYMPTOMS	RATE				
	Very Poor	Poor	Fair	Good	Excellent
	○	○	○	○	○
	○	○	○	○	○
	○	○	○	○	○
	○	○	○	○	○
	○	○	○	○	○

NOTES

257

Daily routine

___ / ___ / ___

M	T	W	T	F	S	S
●	●	●	●	●	●	●

OUTSIDE TIME

TIME	LENGTH

BATHROOM TIME

		wet	b.m.
		wet	b.m.
		wet	b.m.
		wet	b.m.

SLEEP TIME

TIME	LENGTH

Snacks

MY DAY WAS

○ **Good**   ○ **Fair**   ○ **Poor**

Meals

Morning	○ **Good**	○ **Fair**	○ **Poor**
Evening	○ **Good**	○ **Fair**	○ **Poor**

DAILY GOALS

ACTIVITY	LENGTH	MEDICINE	TIME	DOSAGE

SEXUAL HEALTH

SYMPTOMS	RATE				
	Very Poor	Poor	Fair	Good	Excellent
	○	○	○	○	○
	○	○	○	○	○
	○	○	○	○	○
	○	○	○	○	○
	○	○	○	○	○

NOTES

Daily routine

_____ / _____ / _____

M	T	W	T	F	S	S
•	•	•	•	•	•	•

OUTSIDE TIME

TIME	LENGTH

BATHROOM TIME

	wet	b.m.
	wet	b.m.
	wet	b.m.
	wet	b.m.

SLEEP TIME

TIME	LENGTH

Snacks

MY DAY WAS

○ **Good**   ○ **Fair**   ○ **Poor**

Meals

Morning	○ **Good**	○ **Fair**	○ **Poor**
Evening	○ **Good**	○ **Fair**	○ **Poor**

DAILY GOALS

ACTIVITY	LENGTH	MEDICINE	TIME	DOSAGE

SEXUAL HEALTH

SYMPTOMS	RATE				
	Very Poor	**Poor**	**Fair**	**Good**	**Excellent**
	○	○	○	○	○
	○	○	○	○	○
	○	○	○	○	○
	○	○	○	○	○
	○	○	○	○	○

NOTES

259

Daily routine

___ ___ / ___ / ___

M T W T F S S

OUTSIDE TIME

TIME	LENGTH

BATHROOM TIME

	wet	b.m.
	wet	b.m.
	wet	b.m.
	wet	b.m.

SLEEP TIME

TIME	LENGTH

Snacks

MY DAY WAS

○ Good   ○ Fair   ○ Poor

Meals

Morning	○ Good	○ Fair	○ Poor
Evening	○ Good	○ Fair	○ Poor

DAILY GOALS

ACTIVITY	LENGTH	MEDICINE	TIME	DOSAGE

SEXUAL HEALTH

SYMPTOMS	RATE				
	Very Poor	Poor	Fair	Good	Excellent
	○	○	○	○	○
	○	○	○	○	○
	○	○	○	○	○
	○	○	○	○	○
	○	○	○	○	○

NOTES

Daily routine

____ / ____ / ____

	M	T	W	T	F	S	S
	●	●	●	●	●	●	●

OUTSIDE TIME

TIME	LENGTH

BATHROOM TIME

	wet	b.m.
	wet	b.m.
	wet	b.m.
	wet	b.m.

SLEEP TIME

TIME	LENGTH

Snacks

MY DAY WAS

○ **Good**   ○ **Fair**   ○ **Poor**

Meals

Morning	○ Good	○ Fair	○ Poor
Evening	○ Good	○ Fair	○ Poor

DAILY GOALS

ACTIVITY	LENGTH	MEDICINE	TIME	DOSAGE

SEXUAL HEALTH

SYMPTOMS	RATE				
	Very Poor	Poor	Fair	Good	Excellent
	○	○	○	○	○
	○	○	○	○	○
	○	○	○	○	○
	○	○	○	○	○
	○	○	○	○	○

NOTES

261

Daily routine

___ / ___ / ___

M	T	W	T	F	S	S
●	●	●	●	●	●	●

OUTSIDE TIME

TIME	LENGTH

BATHROOM TIME

		wet	b.m.
		wet	b.m.
		wet	b.m.
		wet	b.m.

SLEEP TIME

TIME	LENGTH

Snacks

MY DAY WAS

○ **Good** ○ **Fair** ○ **Poor**

Meals

Morning	○ Good	○ Fair	○ Poor
Evening	○ Good	○ Fair	○ Poor

DAILY GOALS

ACTIVITY	LENGTH	MEDICINE	TIME	DOSAGE

SEXUAL HEALTH

SYMPTOMS	RATE				
	Very Poor	Poor	Fair	Good	Excellent
	○	○	○	○	○
	○	○	○	○	○
	○	○	○	○	○
	○	○	○	○	○
	○	○	○	○	○

NOTES

Daily routine

____ / ____ / ____

M	T	W	T	F	S	S
●	●	●	●	●	●	●

OUTSIDE TIME

TIME	LENGTH

BATHROOM TIME

	wet	b.m.
	wet	b.m.
	wet	b.m.
	wet	b.m.

SLEEP TIME

TIME	LENGTH

Snacks

MY DAY WAS

○ **Good** ○ **Fair** ○ **Poor**

Meals

Morning	○ Good	○ Fair	○ Poor
Evening	○ Good	○ Fair	○ Poor

DAILY GOALS

ACTIVITY	LENGTH	MEDICINE	TIME	DOSAGE

SEXUAL HEALTH

SYMPTOMS	RATE				
	Very Poor	Poor	Fair	Good	Excellent
	○	○	○	○	○
	○	○	○	○	○
	○	○	○	○	○
	○	○	○	○	○
	○	○	○	○	○

NOTES

Daily routine

___ / ___ / ___

M T W T F S S

OUTSIDE TIME

TIME	LENGTH

BATHROOM TIME

	wet	b.m.
	wet	b.m.
	wet	b.m.
	wet	b.m.

SLEEP TIME

TIME	LENGTH

Snacks

MY DAY WAS

○ **Good**   ○ **Fair**   ○ **Poor**

Meals

Morning	○ Good	○ Fair	○ Poor
Evening	○ Good	○ Fair	○ Poor

DAILY GOALS

ACTIVITY	LENGTH	MEDICINE	TIME	DOSAGE

SEXUAL HEALTH

SYMPTOMS	RATE				
	Very Poor	Poor	Fair	Good	Excellent
	○	○	○	○	○
	○	○	○	○	○
	○	○	○	○	○
	○	○	○	○	○
	○	○	○	○	○

NOTES

Daily routine

___ / ___ / ___

M T W T F S S

OUTSIDE TIME

TIME	LENGTH

BATHROOM TIME

	wet	b.m.
	wet	b.m.
	wet	b.m.
	wet	b.m.

SLEEP TIME

TIME	LENGTH

Snacks

MY DAY WAS

○ Good   ○ Fair   ○ Poor

Meals

Morning	○ Good	○ Fair	○ Poor
Evening	○ Good	○ Fair	○ Poor

DAILY GOALS

ACTIVITY	LENGTH	MEDICINE	TIME	DOSAGE

SEXUAL HEALTH

SYMPTOMS	RATE				
	Very Poor	Poor	Fair	Good	Excellent
	○	○	○	○	○
	○	○	○	○	○
	○	○	○	○	○
	○	○	○	○	○
	○	○	○	○	○

NOTES

Daily routine

___ / ___ / ___

| M | T | W | T | F | S | S |

OUTSIDE TIME

TIME	LENGTH

BATHROOM TIME

	wet	b.m.
	wet	b.m.
	wet	b.m.
	wet	b.m.

SLEEP TIME

TIME	LENGTH

Snacks

MY DAY WAS
○ Good ○ Fair ○ Poor

Meals
Morning ○ Good ○ Fair ○ Poor
Evening ○ Good ○ Fair ○ Poor

DAILY GOALS

ACTIVITY	LENGTH	MEDICINE	TIME	DOSAGE

SEXUAL HEALTH

SYMPTOMS	Very Poor	Poor	Fair	Good	Excellent
	O	O	O	O	O
	O	O	O	O	O
	O	O	O	O	O
	O	O	O	O	O
	O	O	O	O	O

RATE

NOTES

Daily routine

_____ / _____ / _____

M T W T F S S

OUTSIDE TIME

TIME	LENGTH

BATHROOM TIME

	wet	b.m.
	wet	b.m.
	wet	b.m.
	wet	b.m.

SLEEP TIME

TIME	LENGTH

Snacks

MY DAY WAS

○ **Good**   ○ **Fair**   ○ **Poor**

Meals

Morning   ○ **Good**   ○ **Fair**   ○ **Poor**

Evening   ○ **Good**   ○ **Fair**   ○ **Poor**

DAILY GOALS

ACTIVITY	LENGTH	MEDICINE	TIME	DOSAGE

SEXUAL HEALTH

SYMPTOMS	RATE				
	Very Poor	Poor	Fair	Good	Excellent
	○	○	○	○	○
	○	○	○	○	○
	○	○	○	○	○
	○	○	○	○	○
	○	○	○	○	○

NOTES

267

Daily routine

____ / ____ / ____

M	T	W	T	F	S	S
●	●	●	●	●	●	●

OUTSIDE TIME

TIME	LENGTH

BATHROOM TIME

	wet	b.m.
	wet	b.m.
	wet	b.m.
	wet	b.m.

SLEEP TIME

TIME	LENGTH

Snacks

MY DAY WAS

○ Good   ○ Fair   ○ Poor

Meals

Morning	○ Good	○ Fair	○ Poor
Evening	○ Good	○ Fair	○ Poor

DAILY GOALS

ACTIVITY	LENGTH	MEDICINE	TIME	DOSAGE

SEXUAL HEALTH

SYMPTOMS	RATE				
	Very Poor	Poor	Fair	Good	Excellent
	○	○	○	○	○
	○	○	○	○	○
	○	○	○	○	○
	○	○	○	○	○
	○	○	○	○	○

NOTES

Daily routine

____ / ____ / ____

M T W T F S S

OUTSIDE TIME

TIME	LENGTH

BATHROOM TIME

	wet	b.m.
	wet	b.m.
	wet	b.m.
	wet	b.m.

SLEEP TIME

TIME	LENGTH

Snacks

MY DAY WAS

○ Good   ○ Fair   ○ Poor

Meals

Morning	○ Good	○ Fair	○ Poor
Evening	○ Good	○ Fair	○ Poor

DAILY GOALS

ACTIVITY	LENGTH	MEDICINE	TIME	DOSAGE

SEXUAL HEALTH

SYMPTOMS	RATE				
	Very Poor	Poor	Fair	Good	Excellent
	○	○	○	○	○
	○	○	○	○	○
	○	○	○	○	○
	○	○	○	○	○
	○	○	○	○	○

NOTES

Daily routine

____ / ____ / ____

| M | T | W | T | F | S | S |

OUTSIDE TIME

TIME	LENGTH

BATHROOM TIME

	wet	b.m.
	wet	b.m.
	wet	b.m.
	wet	b.m.

SLEEP TIME

TIME	LENGTH

Snacks

MY DAY WAS

○ Good   ○ Fair   ○ Poor

Meals

| Morning | ○ Good | ○ Fair | ○ Poor |
| Evening | ○ Good | ○ Fair | ○ Poor |

DAILY GOALS

ACTIVITY	LENGTH	MEDICINE	TIME	DOSAGE

SEXUAL HEALTH

SYMPTOMS	RATE				
	Very Poor	Poor	Fair	Good	Excellent
	○	○	○	○	○
	○	○	○	○	○
	○	○	○	○	○
	○	○	○	○	○
	○	○	○	○	○

NOTES

Daily routine

____ / ____ / ____

M	T	W	T	F	S	S
●	●	●	●	●	●	●

OUTSIDE TIME

TIME	LENGTH

BATHROOM TIME

	wet	b.m.
	wet	b.m.
	wet	b.m.
	wet	b.m.

SLEEP TIME

TIME	LENGTH

Snacks

MY DAY WAS

○ **Good** ○ **Fair** ○ **Poor**

Meals

Morning	○ **Good**	○ **Fair**	○ **Poor**
Evening	○ **Good**	○ **Fair**	○ **Poor**

DAILY GOALS

ACTIVITY	LENGTH	MEDICINE	TIME	DOSAGE

SEXUAL HEALTH

SYMPTOMS	RATE				
	Very Poor	Poor	Fair	Good	Excellent
	○	○	○	○	○
	○	○	○	○	○
	○	○	○	○	○
	○	○	○	○	○
	○	○	○	○	○

NOTES

271

Daily routine

____ / ____ / ____

M T W T F S S

OUTSIDE TIME

TIME	LENGTH

BATHROOM TIME

	wet	b.m.
	wet	b.m.
	wet	b.m.
	wet	b.m.

SLEEP TIME

TIME	LENGTH

Snacks

MY DAY WAS

○ Good   ○ Fair   ○ Poor

Meals

Morning	○ Good	○ Fair	○ Poor
Evening	○ Good	○ Fair	○ Poor

DAILY GOALS

ACTIVITY	LENGTH	MEDICINE	TIME	DOSAGE

SEXUAL HEALTH

SYMPTOMS	RATE				
	Very Poor	Poor	Fair	Good	Excellent
	○	○	○	○	○
	○	○	○	○	○
	○	○	○	○	○
	○	○	○	○	○
	○	○	○	○	○

NOTES

Daily routine

____ / ____ / ____

M	T	W	T	F	S	S
●	●	●	●	●	●	●

OUTSIDE TIME

TIME	LENGTH

BATHROOM TIME

	wet	b.m.
	wet	b.m.
	wet	b.m.
	wet	b.m.

SLEEP TIME

TIME	LENGTH

Snacks

MY DAY WAS

○ Good   ○ Fair   ○ Poor

Meals

Morning	○ Good	○ Fair	○ Poor
Evening	○ Good	○ Fair	○ Poor

DAILY GOALS

ACTIVITY	LENGTH	MEDICINE	TIME	DOSAGE

SEXUAL HEALTH

SYMPTOMS	RATE				
	Very Poor	Poor	Fair	Good	Excellent
	○	○	○	○	○
	○	○	○	○	○
	○	○	○	○	○
	○	○	○	○	○
	○	○	○	○	○

NOTES

Daily routine

___ / ___ / ___

| M | T | W | T | F | S | S |

OUTSIDE TIME

TIME	LENGTH

BATHROOM TIME

	wet	b.m.
	wet	b.m.
	wet	b.m.
	wet	b.m.

SLEEP TIME

TIME	LENGTH

Snacks

MY DAY WAS

○ **Good**   ○ **Fair**   ○ **Poor**

Meals

Morning	○ Good	○ Fair	○ Poor
Evening	○ Good	○ Fair	○ Poor

DAILY GOALS

ACTIVITY	LENGTH	MEDICINE	TIME	DOSAGE

SEXUAL HEALTH

SYMPTOMS	RATE				
	Very Poor	Poor	Fair	Good	Excellent
	○	○	○	○	○
	○	○	○	○	○
	○	○	○	○	○
	○	○	○	○	○
	○	○	○	○	○

NOTES

Daily routine

___ / ___ / ___

	M	T	W	T	F	S	S
	•	•	•	•	•	•	•

OUTSIDE TIME

TIME	LENGTH

BATHROOM TIME

	wet	b.m.
	wet	b.m.
	wet	b.m.
	wet	b.m.

SLEEP TIME

TIME	LENGTH

Snacks

MY DAY WAS

○ **Good**   ○ **Fair**   ○ **Poor**

Meals

Morning	○ **Good**	○ **Fair**	○ **Poor**
Evening	○ **Good**	○ **Fair**	○ **Poor**

DAILY GOALS

ACTIVITY	LENGTH	MEDICINE	TIME	DOSAGE

SEXUAL HEALTH

SYMPTOMS	RATE				
	Very Poor	Poor	Fair	Good	Excellent
	○	○	○	○	○
	○	○	○	○	○
	○	○	○	○	○
	○	○	○	○	○
	○	○	○	○	○

NOTES

Daily routine

___ / ___ / ___

M	T	W	T	F	S	S
●	●	●	●	●	●	●

OUTSIDE TIME

TIME	LENGTH

BATHROOM TIME

	wet	b.m.
	wet	b.m.
	wet	b.m.
	wet	b.m.

SLEEP TIME

TIME	LENGTH

Snacks

MY DAY WAS

○ Good   ○ Fair   ○ Poor

Meals

Morning	○ Good	○ Fair	○ Poor
Evening	○ Good	○ Fair	○ Poor

DAILY GOALS

ACTIVITY	LENGTH	MEDICINE	TIME	DOSAGE

SEXUAL HEALTH

SYMPTOMS	RATE				
	Very Poor	Poor	Fair	Good	Excellent
	○	○	○	○	○
	○	○	○	○	○
	○	○	○	○	○
	○	○	○	○	○
	○	○	○	○	○

NOTES

Daily routine

____ / ____ / ____

M	T	W	T	F	S	S
●	●	●	●	●	●	●

OUTSIDE TIME

TIME	LENGTH

BATHROOM TIME

		wet	b.m.
		wet	b.m.
		wet	b.m.
		wet	b.m.

SLEEP TIME

TIME	LENGTH

Snacks

MY DAY WAS

○ **Good**   ○ **Fair**   ○ **Poor**

Meals

Morning	○ **Good**	○ **Fair**	○ **Poor**
Evening	○ **Good**	○ **Fair**	○ **Poor**

DAILY GOALS

ACTIVITY	LENGTH	MEDICINE	TIME	DOSAGE

SEXUAL HEALTH

SYMPTOMS	RATE				
	Very Poor	Poor	Fair	Good	Excellent
	○	○	○	○	○
	○	○	○	○	○
	○	○	○	○	○
	○	○	○	○	○
	○	○	○	○	○

NOTES

277

Daily routine

____ / ____ / ____

M	T	W	T	F	S	S
●	●	●	●	●	●	●

OUTSIDE TIME

TIME	LENGTH

BATHROOM TIME

	wet	b.m.
	wet	b.m.
	wet	b.m.
	wet	b.m.

SLEEP TIME

TIME	LENGTH

Snacks

MY DAY WAS

○ **Good**　　○ **Fair**　　○ **Poor**

Meals

Morning	○ Good	○ Fair	○ Poor
Evening	○ Good	○ Fair	○ Poor

DAILY GOALS

ACTIVITY	LENGTH	MEDICINE	TIME	DOSAGE

SEXUAL HEALTH

SYMPTOMS	RATE				
	Very Poor	Poor	Fair	Good	Excellent
	○	○	○	○	○
	○	○	○	○	○
	○	○	○	○	○
	○	○	○	○	○
	○	○	○	○	○

NOTES

Daily routine

___ / ___ / ___

M	T	W	T	F	S	S
•	•	•	•	•	•	•

OUTSIDE TIME

TIME	LENGTH

BATHROOM TIME

	wet	b.m.
	wet	b.m.
	wet	b.m.
	wet	b.m.

SLEEP TIME

TIME	LENGTH

Snacks

MY DAY WAS

○ **Good**   ○ **Fair**   ○ **Poor**

Meals

Morning	○ **Good**	○ **Fair**	○ **Poor**
Evening	○ **Good**	○ **Fair**	○ **Poor**

DAILY GOALS

ACTIVITY	LENGTH	MEDICINE	TIME	DOSAGE

SEXUAL HEALTH

SYMPTOMS	RATE				
	Very Poor	Poor	Fair	Good	Excellent
	○	○	○	○	○
	○	○	○	○	○
	○	○	○	○	○
	○	○	○	○	○
	○	○	○	○	○

NOTES

Daily routine

____ / ____ / ____

M	T	W	T	F	S	S

OUTSIDE TIME

TIME	LENGTH

BATHROOM TIME

	wet	b.m.
	wet	b.m.
	wet	b.m.
	wet	b.m.

SLEEP TIME

TIME	LENGTH

Snacks

MY DAY WAS

○ Good   ○ Fair   ○ Poor

Meals

Morning	○ Good	○ Fair	○ Poor
Evening	○ Good	○ Fair	○ Poor

DAILY GOALS

ACTIVITY	LENGTH	MEDICINE	TIME	DOSAGE

SEXUAL HEALTH

SYMPTOMS	RATE				
	Very Poor	Poor	Fair	Good	Excellent
	○	○	○	○	○
	○	○	○	○	○
	○	○	○	○	○
	○	○	○	○	○
	○	○	○	○	○

NOTES

Daily routine

____ / ____ / ____

M	T	W	T	F	S	S
•	•	•	•	•	•	•

OUTSIDE TIME

TIME	LENGTH

BATHROOM TIME

	wet	b.m.
	wet	b.m.
	wet	b.m.
	wet	b.m.

SLEEP TIME

TIME	LENGTH

Snacks

MY DAY WAS

○ **Good**   ○ **Fair**   ○ **Poor**

Meals

Morning	○ Good	○ Fair	○ Poor
Evening	○ Good	○ Fair	○ Poor

DAILY GOALS

ACTIVITY	LENGTH	MEDICINE	TIME	DOSAGE

SEXUAL HEALTH

SYMPTOMS	RATE				
	Very Poor	Poor	Fair	Good	Excellent
	○	○	○	○	○
	○	○	○	○	○
	○	○	○	○	○
	○	○	○	○	○
	○	○	○	○	○

NOTES

Daily routine

____ / ____ / ____

M	T	W	T	F	S	S
●	●	●	●	●	●	●

OUTSIDE TIME

TIME	LENGTH

BATHROOM TIME

	wet	b.m.
	wet	b.m.
	wet	b.m.
	wet	b.m.

SLEEP TIME

TIME	LENGTH

Snacks

MY DAY WAS

○ **Good**   ○ **Fair**   ○ **Poor**

Meals

Morning	○ **Good**	○ **Fair**	○ **Poor**
Evening	○ **Good**	○ **Fair**	○ **Poor**

DAILY GOALS

ACTIVITY	LENGTH	MEDICINE	TIME	DOSAGE

SEXUAL HEALTH

SYMPTOMS	RATE				
	Very Poor	Poor	Fair	Good	Excellent
	○	○	○	○	○
	○	○	○	○	○
	○	○	○	○	○
	○	○	○	○	○
	○	○	○	○	○

NOTES

Daily routine

___ / ___ / ___

M	T	W	T	F	S	S
●	●	●	●	●	●	●

OUTSIDE TIME

TIME	LENGTH

BATHROOM TIME

	wet	b.m.
	wet	b.m.
	wet	b.m.
	wet	b.m.

SLEEP TIME

TIME	LENGTH

Snacks

MY DAY WAS

○ **Good**   ○ **Fair**   ○ **Poor**

Meals

Morning	○ **Good**	○ **Fair**	○ **Poor**
Evening	○ **Good**	○ **Fair**	○ **Poor**

DAILY GOALS

ACTIVITY	LENGTH	MEDICINE	TIME	DOSAGE

SEXUAL HEALTH

SYMPTOMS	RATE				
	Very Poor	Poor	Fair	Good	Excellent
	○	○	○	○	○
	○	○	○	○	○
	○	○	○	○	○
	○	○	○	○	○
	○	○	○	○	○

NOTES

Daily routine

___ / ___ / ___

M	T	W	T	F	S	S
●	●	●	●	●	●	●

OUTSIDE TIME

TIME	LENGTH

BATHROOM TIME

	wet	b.m.
	wet	b.m.
	wet	b.m.
	wet	b.m.

SLEEP TIME

TIME	LENGTH

Snacks

MY DAY WAS

○ Good   ○ Fair   ○ Poor

Meals

Morning	○ Good	○ Fair	○ Poor
Evening	○ Good	○ Fair	○ Poor

DAILY GOALS

ACTIVITY	LENGTH	MEDICINE	TIME	DOSAGE

SEXUAL HEALTH

SYMPTOMS	RATE				
	Very Poor	Poor	Fair	Good	Excellent
	○	○	○	○	○
	○	○	○	○	○
	○	○	○	○	○
	○	○	○	○	○
	○	○	○	○	○

NOTES

Daily routine

____ / ____ / ____

M	T	W	T	F	S	S
●	●	●	●	●	●	●

OUTSIDE TIME

TIME	LENGTH

BATHROOM TIME

		wet	b.m.
		wet	b.m.
		wet	b.m.
		wet	b.m.

SLEEP TIME

TIME	LENGTH

Snacks

MY DAY WAS

○ Good   ○ Fair   ○ Poor

Meals

Morning	○ Good	○ Fair	○ Poor
Evening	○ Good	○ Fair	○ Poor

DAILY GOALS

ACTIVITY	LENGTH	MEDICINE	TIME	DOSAGE

SEXUAL HEALTH

SYMPTOMS	RATE				
	Very Poor	Poor	Fair	Good	Excellent
	○	○	○	○	○
	○	○	○	○	○
	○	○	○	○	○
	○	○	○	○	○
	○	○	○	○	○

NOTES

Daily routine

____ / ____ / ____

M   T   W   T   F   S   S

OUTSIDE TIME

TIME	LENGTH

BATHROOM TIME

	wet	b.m.
	wet	b.m.
	wet	b.m.
	wet	b.m.

SLEEP TIME

TIME	LENGTH

Snacks

MY DAY WAS

○ **Good**   ○ **Fair**   ○ **Poor**

Meals

Morning	○ Good	○ Fair	○ Poor
Evening	○ Good	○ Fair	○ Poor

DAILY GOALS

ACTIVITY	LENGTH	MEDICINE	TIME	DOSAGE

SEXUAL HEALTH

SYMPTOMS	RATE				
	Very Poor	Poor	Fair	Good	Excellent
	○	○	○	○	○
	○	○	○	○	○
	○	○	○	○	○
	○	○	○	○	○
	○	○	○	○	○

NOTES

Daily routine

___ / ___ / ___

M T W T F S S

OUTSIDE TIME

TIME	LENGTH

BATHROOM TIME

		wet	b.m.
		wet	b.m.
		wet	b.m.
		wet	b.m.

SLEEP TIME

TIME	LENGTH

Snacks

MY DAY WAS

○ Good   ○ Fair   ○ Poor

Meals

Morning	○ Good	○ Fair	○ Poor
Evening	○ Good	○ Fair	○ Poor

DAILY GOALS

ACTIVITY	LENGTH	MEDICINE	TIME	DOSAGE

SEXUAL HEALTH

SYMPTOMS	RATE				
	Very Poor	Poor	Fair	Good	Excellent
	○	○	○	○	○
	○	○	○	○	○
	○	○	○	○	○
	○	○	○	○	○
	○	○	○	○	○

NOTES

Daily routine

____ / ____ / ____

M	T	W	T	F	S	S
●	●	●	●	●	●	●

OUTSIDE TIME

TIME	LENGTH

BATHROOM TIME

	wet	b.m.
	wet	b.m.
	wet	b.m.
	wet	b.m.

SLEEP TIME

TIME	LENGTH

Snacks

MY DAY WAS

○ **Good**   ○ **Fair**   ○ **Poor**

Meals

Morning	○ **Good**	○ **Fair**	○ **Poor**
Evening	○ **Good**	○ **Fair**	○ **Poor**

DAILY GOALS

ACTIVITY	LENGTH	MEDICINE	TIME	DOSAGE

SEXUAL HEALTH

SYMPTOMS	RATE				
	Very Poor	Poor	Fair	Good	Excellent
	○	○	○	○	○
	○	○	○	○	○
	○	○	○	○	○
	○	○	○	○	○
	○	○	○	○	○

NOTES

Daily routine

___ / ___ / ___

| M | T | W | T | F | S | S |

OUTSIDE TIME

TIME	LENGTH

BATHROOM TIME

	wet	b.m.
	wet	b.m.
	wet	b.m.
	wet	b.m.

SLEEP TIME

TIME	LENGTH

Snacks

MY DAY WAS

○ Good   ○ Fair   ○ Poor

Meals

Morning	○ Good	○ Fair	○ Poor
Evening	○ Good	○ Fair	○ Poor

DAILY GOALS

ACTIVITY	LENGTH	MEDICINE	TIME	DOSAGE

SEXUAL HEALTH

SYMPTOMS	RATE				
	Very Poor	Poor	Fair	Good	Excellent
	○	○	○	○	○
	○	○	○	○	○
	○	○	○	○	○
	○	○	○	○	○
	○	○	○	○	○

NOTES

Daily routine

___ / ___ / ___

M	T	W	T	F	S	S
●	●	●	●	●	●	●

OUTSIDE TIME

TIME	LENGTH

BATHROOM TIME

	wet	b.m.
	wet	b.m.
	wet	b.m.
	wet	b.m.

SLEEP TIME

TIME	LENGTH

Snacks

MY DAY WAS

○ Good   ○ Fair   ○ Poor

Meals

Morning	○ Good	○ Fair	○ Poor
Evening	○ Good	○ Fair	○ Poor

DAILY GOALS

ACTIVITY	LENGTH	MEDICINE	TIME	DOSAGE

SEXUAL HEALTH

SYMPTOMS	RATE				
	Very Poor	Poor	Fair	Good	Excellent
	○	○	○	○	○
	○	○	○	○	○
	○	○	○	○	○
	○	○	○	○	○
	○	○	○	○	○

NOTES

Daily routine

____ / ____ / ____

M T W T F S S
● ● ● ● ● ● ●

OUTSIDE TIME

TIME	LENGTH

BATHROOM TIME

	wet	b.m.
	wet	b.m.
	wet	b.m.
	wet	b.m.

SLEEP TIME

TIME	LENGTH

Snacks

MY DAY WAS

○ Good   ○ Fair   ○ Poor

Meals

Morning	○ Good	○ Fair	○ Poor
Evening	○ Good	○ Fair	○ Poor

DAILY GOALS

ACTIVITY	LENGTH	MEDICINE	TIME	DOSAGE

SEXUAL HEALTH

SYMPTOMS	RATE				
	Very Poor	Poor	Fair	Good	Excellent
	○	○	○	○	○
	○	○	○	○	○
	○	○	○	○	○
	○	○	○	○	○
	○	○	○	○	○

NOTES

Daily routine

____ / ____ / ____

M	T	W	T	F	S	S
●	●	●	●	●	●	●

OUTSIDE TIME

TIME	LENGTH

BATHROOM TIME

	wet	b.m.
	wet	b.m.
	wet	b.m.
	wet	b.m.

SLEEP TIME

TIME	LENGTH

Snacks

MY DAY WAS

○ Good   ○ Fair   ○ Poor

Meals

Morning	○ Good	○ Fair	○ Poor
Evening	○ Good	○ Fair	○ Poor

DAILY GOALS

ACTIVITY	LENGTH	MEDICINE	TIME	DOSAGE

SEXUAL HEALTH

SYMPTOMS	RATE				
	Very Poor	Poor	Fair	Good	Excellent
	○	○	○	○	○
	○	○	○	○	○
	○	○	○	○	○
	○	○	○	○	○
	○	○	○	○	○

NOTES

Daily routine

___ / ___ / ___

M	T	W	T	F	S	S
●	●	●	●	●	●	●

OUTSIDE TIME

TIME	LENGTH

BATHROOM TIME

	wet	b.m.
	wet	b.m.
	wet	b.m.
	wet	b.m.

SLEEP TIME

TIME	LENGTH

Snacks

MY DAY WAS

○ Good   ○ Fair   ○ Poor

Meals

Morning	○ Good	○ Fair	○ Poor
Evening	○ Good	○ Fair	○ Poor

DAILY GOALS

ACTIVITY	LENGTH	MEDICINE	TIME	DOSAGE

SEXUAL HEALTH

SYMPTOMS	RATE				
	Very Poor	Poor	Fair	Good	Excellent
	○	○	○	○	○
	○	○	○	○	○
	○	○	○	○	○
	○	○	○	○	○
	○	○	○	○	○

NOTES

293

Daily routine

_____ / _____ / _____

M   T   W   T   F   S   S
●   ●   ●   ●   ●   ●   ●

OUTSIDE TIME

TIME	LENGTH

BATHROOM TIME

	wet	b.m.
	wet	b.m.
	wet	b.m.
	wet	b.m.

SLEEP TIME

TIME	LENGTH

Snacks

MY DAY WAS

○ **Good**   ○ **Fair**   ○ **Poor**

Meals

Morning	○ **Good**	○ **Fair**	○ **Poor**
Evening	○ **Good**	○ **Fair**	○ **Poor**

DAILY GOALS

ACTIVITY	LENGTH	MEDICINE	TIME	DOSAGE

SEXUAL HEALTH

SYMPTOMS	RATE				
	Very Poor	Poor	Fair	Good	Excellent
	○	○	○	○	○
	○	○	○	○	○
	○	○	○	○	○
	○	○	○	○	○
	○	○	○	○	○

NOTES

Daily routine

____ / ____ / ____

M	T	W	T	F	S	S
●	●	●	●	●	●	●

OUTSIDE TIME

TIME	LENGTH

BATHROOM TIME

	wet	b.m.
	wet	b.m.
	wet	b.m.
	wet	b.m.

SLEEP TIME

TIME	LENGTH

Snacks

MY DAY WAS

○ **Good**   ○ **Fair**   ○ **Poor**

Meals

Morning	○ **Good**	○ **Fair**	○ **Poor**
Evening	○ **Good**	○ **Fair**	○ **Poor**

DAILY GOALS

ACTIVITY	LENGTH	MEDICINE	TIME	DOSAGE

SEXUAL HEALTH

SYMPTOMS	RATE				
	Very Poor	Poor	Fair	Good	Excellent
	○	○	○	○	○
	○	○	○	○	○
	○	○	○	○	○
	○	○	○	○	○
	○	○	○	○	○

NOTES

Daily routine

____ / ____ / ____

M	T	W	T	F	S	S
●	●	●	●	●	●	●

OUTSIDE TIME

TIME	LENGTH

BATHROOM TIME

	wet	b.m.
	wet	b.m.
	wet	b.m.
	wet	b.m.

SLEEP TIME

TIME	LENGTH

Snacks

MY DAY WAS

○ Good   ○ Fair   ○ Poor

Meals

Morning	○ Good	○ Fair	○ Poor
Evening	○ Good	○ Fair	○ Poor

DAILY GOALS

ACTIVITY	LENGTH	MEDICINE	TIME	DOSAGE

SEXUAL HEALTH

SYMPTOMS	RATE				
	Very Poor	Poor	Fair	Good	Excellent
	○	○	○	○	○
	○	○	○	○	○
	○	○	○	○	○
	○	○	○	○	○
	○	○	○	○	○

NOTES

Daily routine

_____ / _____ / _____

M	T	W	T	F	S	S
●	●	●	●	●	●	●

OUTSIDE TIME

TIME	LENGTH

BATHROOM TIME

	wet	b.m.
	wet	b.m.
	wet	b.m.
	wet	b.m.

SLEEP TIME

TIME	LENGTH

Snacks

MY DAY WAS

○ Good   ○ Fair   ○ Poor

Meals

Morning	○ Good	○ Fair	○ Poor
Evening	○ Good	○ Fair	○ Poor

DAILY GOALS

ACTIVITY	LENGTH	MEDICINE	TIME	DOSAGE

SEXUAL HEALTH

SYMPTOMS	RATE				
	Very Poor	Poor	Fair	Good	Excellent
	○	○	○	○	○
	○	○	○	○	○
	○	○	○	○	○
	○	○	○	○	○
	○	○	○	○	○

NOTES

Daily routine

___ / ___ / ___

| M | T | W | T | F | S | S |

OUTSIDE TIME

TIME	LENGTH

BATHROOM TIME

	wet	b.m.
	wet	b.m.
	wet	b.m.
	wet	b.m.

SLEEP TIME

TIME	LENGTH

Snacks

MY DAY WAS

○ Good   ○ Fair   ○ Poor

Meals

| Morning | ○ Good | ○ Fair | ○ Poor |
| Evening | ○ Good | ○ Fair | ○ Poor |

DAILY GOALS

ACTIVITY	LENGTH	MEDICINE	TIME	DOSAGE

SEXUAL HEALTH

SYMPTOMS	RATE				
	Very Poor	Poor	Fair	Good	Excellent
	○	○	○	○	○
	○	○	○	○	○
	○	○	○	○	○
	○	○	○	○	○
	○	○	○	○	○

NOTES

Daily routine

____ / ____ / ____

M	T	W	T	F	S	S
●	●	●	●	●	●	●

OUTSIDE TIME

TIME	LENGTH

BATHROOM TIME

	wet	b.m.
	wet	b.m.
	wet	b.m.
	wet	b.m.

SLEEP TIME

TIME	LENGTH

Snacks

MY DAY WAS

○ **Good**   ○ **Fair**   ○ **Poor**

Meals

Morning	○ Good	○ Fair	○ Poor
Evening	○ Good	○ Fair	○ Poor

DAILY GOALS

ACTIVITY	LENGTH	MEDICINE	TIME	DOSAGE

SEXUAL HEALTH

SYMPTOMS	RATE				
	Very Poor	Poor	Fair	Good	Excellent
	○	○	○	○	○
	○	○	○	○	○
	○	○	○	○	○
	○	○	○	○	○
	○	○	○	○	○

NOTES

Daily routine

____ / ____ / ____

M T W T F S S

OUTSIDE TIME

TIME	LENGTH

BATHROOM TIME

	wet	b.m.
	wet	b.m.
	wet	b.m.
	wet	b.m.

SLEEP TIME

TIME	LENGTH

Snacks

MY DAY WAS

○ Good   ○ Fair   ○ Poor

Meals

Morning	○ Good	○ Fair	○ Poor
Evening	○ Good	○ Fair	○ Poor

DAILY GOALS

ACTIVITY	LENGTH	MEDICINE	TIME	DOSAGE

SEXUAL HEALTH

SYMPTOMS	RATE				
	Very Poor	Poor	Fair	Good	Excellent
	○	○	○	○	○
	○	○	○	○	○
	○	○	○	○	○
	○	○	○	○	○
	○	○	○	○	○

NOTES

Daily routine

____ / ____ / ____

M   T   W   T   F   S   S

OUTSIDE TIME

TIME	LENGTH

BATHROOM TIME

	wet	b.m.
	wet	b.m.
	wet	b.m.
	wet	b.m.

SLEEP TIME

TIME	LENGTH

Snacks

MY DAY WAS

○ **Good**   ○ **Fair**   ○ **Poor**

Meals

Morning	○ Good	○ Fair	○ Poor
Evening	○ Good	○ Fair	○ Poor

DAILY GOALS

ACTIVITY	LENGTH	MEDICINE	TIME	DOSAGE

SEXUAL HEALTH

SYMPTOMS	RATE				
	Very Poor	Poor	Fair	Good	Excellent
	○	○	○	○	○
	○	○	○	○	○
	○	○	○	○	○
	○	○	○	○	○
	○	○	○	○	○

NOTES

301

Daily routine

____ / ____ / ____

M	T	W	T	F	S	S
●	●	●	●	●	●	●

OUTSIDE TIME

TIME	LENGTH

BATHROOM TIME

	wet	b.m.
	wet	b.m.
	wet	b.m.
	wet	b.m.

SLEEP TIME

TIME	LENGTH

Snacks

MY DAY WAS

○ **Good**   ○ **Fair**   ○ **Poor**

Meals

Morning	○ Good	○ Fair	○ Poor
Evening	○ Good	○ Fair	○ Poor

DAILY GOALS

ACTIVITY	LENGTH	MEDICINE	TIME	DOSAGE

SEXUAL HEALTH

SYMPTOMS	RATE				
	Very Poor	Poor	Fair	Good	Excellent
	○	○	○	○	○
	○	○	○	○	○
	○	○	○	○	○
	○	○	○	○	○
	○	○	○	○	○

NOTES

Daily routine

____ / ____ / ____

M	T	W	T	F	S	S
●	●	●	●	●	●	●

OUTSIDE TIME

TIME	LENGTH

BATHROOM TIME

	wet	b.m.
	wet	b.m.
	wet	b.m.
	wet	b.m.

SLEEP TIME

TIME	LENGTH

Snacks

MY DAY WAS

○ **Good**   ○ **Fair**   ○ **Poor**

Meals

Morning   ○ **Good**   ○ **Fair**   ○ **Poor**

Evening   ○ **Good**   ○ **Fair**   ○ **Poor**

DAILY GOALS

ACTIVITY	LENGTH	MEDICINE	TIME	DOSAGE

SEXUAL HEALTH

SYMPTOMS	RATE				
	Very Poor	Poor	Fair	Good	Excellent
	○	○	○	○	○
	○	○	○	○	○
	○	○	○	○	○
	○	○	○	○	○
	○	○	○	○	○

NOTES

303

Daily routine

___ / ___ / ___

OUTSIDE TIME

TIME	LENGTH

BATHROOM TIME

	wet	b.m.
	wet	b.m.
	wet	b.m.
	wet	b.m.

SLEEP TIME

TIME	LENGTH

Snacks

M	T	W	T	F	S	S
●	●	●	●	●	●	●

MY DAY WAS

○ Good   ○ Fair   ○ Poor

Meals

| Morning | ○ Good | ○ Fair | ○ Poor |
| Evening | ○ Good | ○ Fair | ○ Poor |

DAILY GOALS

ACTIVITY	LENGTH	MEDICINE	TIME	DOSAGE

SEXUAL HEALTH

SYMPTOMS	RATE				
	Very Poor	Poor	Fair	Good	Excellent
	○	○	○	○	○
	○	○	○	○	○
	○	○	○	○	○
	○	○	○	○	○
	○	○	○	○	○

NOTES

Daily routine

____ / ____ / ____

M	T	W	T	F	S	S
•	•	•	•	•	•	•

OUTSIDE TIME

TIME	LENGTH

BATHROOM TIME

	wet	b.m.
	wet	b.m.
	wet	b.m.
	wet	b.m.

SLEEP TIME

TIME	LENGTH

Snacks

MY DAY WAS

○ Good   ○ Fair   ○ Poor

Meals

| Morning | ○ Good | ○ Fair | ○ Poor |
| Evening | ○ Good | ○ Fair | ○ Poor |

DAILY GOALS

ACTIVITY	LENGTH	MEDICINE	TIME	DOSAGE

SEXUAL HEALTH

SYMPTOMS	RATE				
	Very Poor	Poor	Fair	Good	Excellent
	○	○	○	○	○
	○	○	○	○	○
	○	○	○	○	○
	○	○	○	○	○
	○	○	○	○	○

NOTES

Daily routine

___ / ___ / ___

M	T	W	T	F	S	S
•	•	•	•	•	•	•

OUTSIDE TIME

TIME	LENGTH

BATHROOM TIME

	wet	b.m.
	wet	b.m.
	wet	b.m.
	wet	b.m.

SLEEP TIME

TIME	LENGTH

Snacks

MY DAY WAS

○ **Good**　　○ **Fair**　　○ **Poor**

Meals

Morning	○ Good	○ Fair	○ Poor
Evening	○ Good	○ Fair	○ Poor

DAILY GOALS

ACTIVITY	LENGTH	MEDICINE	TIME	DOSAGE

SEXUAL HEALTH

SYMPTOMS	RATE				
	Very Poor	Poor	Fair	Good	Excellent
	○	○	○	○	○
	○	○	○	○	○
	○	○	○	○	○
	○	○	○	○	○
	○	○	○	○	○

NOTES

Daily routine

___ / ___ / ___

M T W T F S S

OUTSIDE TIME

TIME	LENGTH

BATHROOM TIME

	wet	b.m.
	wet	b.m.
	wet	b.m.
	wet	b.m.

SLEEP TIME

TIME	LENGTH

Snacks

MY DAY WAS

○ **Good**   ○ **Fair**   ○ **Poor**

Meals

Morning	○ Good	○ Fair	○ Poor
Evening	○ Good	○ Fair	○ Poor

DAILY GOALS

ACTIVITY	LENGTH	MEDICINE	TIME	DOSAGE

SEXUAL HEALTH

SYMPTOMS	Very Poor	Poor	Fair	Good	Excellent
	○	○	○	○	○
	○	○	○	○	○
	○	○	○	○	○
	○	○	○	○	○
	○	○	○	○	○

RATE

NOTES

Daily routine

___ / ___ / ___

M	T	W	T	F	S	S
●	●	●	●	●	●	●

OUTSIDE TIME

TIME	LENGTH

BATHROOM TIME

	wet	b.m.
	wet	b.m.
	wet	b.m.
	wet	b.m.

SLEEP TIME

TIME	LENGTH

Snacks

MY DAY WAS

○ **Good**   ○ **Fair**   ○ **Poor**

Meals

Morning	○ Good	○ Fair	○ Poor
Evening	○ Good	○ Fair	○ Poor

DAILY GOALS

ACTIVITY	LENGTH	MEDICINE	TIME	DOSAGE

SEXUAL HEALTH

SYMPTOMS	RATE				
	Very Poor	**Poor**	**Fair**	**Good**	**Excellent**
	○	○	○	○	○
	○	○	○	○	○
	○	○	○	○	○
	○	○	○	○	○
	○	○	○	○	○

NOTES

Daily routine

____ / ____ / ____

M	T	W	T	F	S	S
●	●	●	●	●	●	●

OUTSIDE TIME

TIME	LENGTH

BATHROOM TIME

	wet	b.m.
	wet	b.m.
	wet	b.m.
	wet	b.m.

SLEEP TIME

TIME	LENGTH

Snacks

MY DAY WAS

○ **Good**   ○ **Fair**   ○ **Poor**

Meals

Morning	○ **Good**	○ **Fair**	○ **Poor**
Evening	○ **Good**	○ **Fair**	○ **Poor**

DAILY GOALS

ACTIVITY	LENGTH	MEDICINE	TIME	DOSAGE

SEXUAL HEALTH

SYMPTOMS	RATE				
	Very Poor	Poor	Fair	Good	Excellent
	○	○	○	○	○
	○	○	○	○	○
	○	○	○	○	○
	○	○	○	○	○
	○	○	○	○	○

NOTES

Daily routine

____ / ____ / ____

M T W T F S S
● ● ● ● ● ● ●

OUTSIDE TIME

TIME	LENGTH

BATHROOM TIME

		wet	b.m.
		wet	b.m.
		wet	b.m.
		wet	b.m.

SLEEP TIME

TIME	LENGTH

Snacks

MY DAY WAS

○ Good   ○ Fair   ○ Poor

Meals

Morning	○ Good	○ Fair	○ Poor
Evening	○ Good	○ Fair	○ Poor

DAILY GOALS

ACTIVITY	LENGTH	MEDICINE	TIME	DOSAGE

SEXUAL HEALTH

SYMPTOMS	RATE				
	Very Poor	Poor	Fair	Good	Excellent
	○	○	○	○	○
	○	○	○	○	○
	○	○	○	○	○
	○	○	○	○	○
	○	○	○	○	○

NOTES

Daily routine

____ / ____ / ____

M	T	W	T	F	S	S
●	●	●	●	●	●	●

OUTSIDE TIME

TIME	LENGTH

BATHROOM TIME

	wet	b.m.
	wet	b.m.
	wet	b.m.
	wet	b.m.

SLEEP TIME

TIME	LENGTH

Snacks

MY DAY WAS

○ **Good**   ○ **Fair**   ○ **Poor**

Meals

| **Morning** | ○ **Good** | ○ **Fair** | ○ **Poor** |
| **Evening** | ○ **Good** | ○ **Fair** | ○ **Poor** |

DAILY GOALS

ACTIVITY	LENGTH	MEDICINE	TIME	DOSAGE

SEXUAL HEALTH

SYMPTOMS	RATE				
	Very Poor	Poor	Fair	Good	Excellent
	○	○	○	○	○
	○	○	○	○	○
	○	○	○	○	○
	○	○	○	○	○
	○	○	○	○	○

NOTES

Daily routine

___ / ___ / ___

M	T	W	T	F	S	S
●	●	●	●	●	●	●

OUTSIDE TIME

TIME	LENGTH

BATHROOM TIME

	wet	b.m.
	wet	b.m.
	wet	b.m.
	wet	b.m.

SLEEP TIME

TIME	LENGTH

Snacks

MY DAY WAS

○ Good   ○ Fair   ○ Poor

Meals

Morning	○ Good	○ Fair	○ Poor
Evening	○ Good	○ Fair	○ Poor

DAILY GOALS

ACTIVITY	LENGTH	MEDICINE	TIME	DOSAGE

SEXUAL HEALTH

SYMPTOMS	RATE				
	Very Poor	Poor	Fair	Good	Excellent
	○	○	○	○	○
	○	○	○	○	○
	○	○	○	○	○
	○	○	○	○	○
	○	○	○	○	○

NOTES

Daily routine

_____ / _____ / _____

M	T	W	T	F	S	S
●	●	●	●	●	●	●

OUTSIDE TIME

TIME	LENGTH

BATHROOM TIME

	wet	b.m.
	wet	b.m.
	wet	b.m.
	wet	b.m.

SLEEP TIME

TIME	LENGTH

Snacks

MY DAY WAS

○ **Good**   ○ **Fair**   ○ **Poor**

Meals

Morning	○ **Good**	○ **Fair**	○ **Poor**
Evening	○ **Good**	○ **Fair**	○ **Poor**

DAILY GOALS

ACTIVITY	LENGTH	MEDICINE	TIME	DOSAGE

SEXUAL HEALTH

SYMPTOMS	RATE				
	Very Poor	Poor	Fair	Good	Excellent
	○	○	○	○	○
	○	○	○	○	○
	○	○	○	○	○
	○	○	○	○	○
	○	○	○	○	○

NOTES

313

Daily routine

___ / ___ / ___

M	T	W	T	F	S	S
●	●	●	●	●	●	●

OUTSIDE TIME

TIME	LENGTH

BATHROOM TIME

	wet	b.m.
	wet	b.m.
	wet	b.m.
	wet	b.m.

SLEEP TIME

TIME	LENGTH

Snacks

MY DAY WAS

○ Good   ○ Fair   ○ Poor

Meals

Morning	○ Good	○ Fair	○ Poor
Evening	○ Good	○ Fair	○ Poor

DAILY GOALS

ACTIVITY	LENGTH	MEDICINE	TIME	DOSAGE

SEXUAL HEALTH

SYMPTOMS	RATE				
	Very Poor	Poor	Fair	Good	Excellent
	○	○	○	○	○
	○	○	○	○	○
	○	○	○	○	○
	○	○	○	○	○
	○	○	○	○	○

NOTES

Daily routine

____ / ____ / ____

M	T	W	T	F	S	S
●	●	●	●	●	●	●

OUTSIDE TIME

TIME	LENGTH

BATHROOM TIME

	wet	b.m.
	wet	b.m.
	wet	b.m.
	wet	b.m.

SLEEP TIME

TIME	LENGTH

Snacks

MY DAY WAS

○ **Good**   ○ **Fair**   ○ **Poor**

Meals

Morning	○ **Good**	○ **Fair**	○ **Poor**
Evening	○ **Good**	○ **Fair**	○ **Poor**

DAILY GOALS

ACTIVITY	LENGTH	MEDICINE	TIME	DOSAGE

SEXUAL HEALTH

SYMPTOMS	RATE				
	Very Poor	Poor	Fair	Good	Excellent
	○	○	○	○	○
	○	○	○	○	○
	○	○	○	○	○
	○	○	○	○	○
	○	○	○	○	○

NOTES

Daily routine

____ / ____ / ____

M T W T F S S

OUTSIDE TIME

TIME	LENGTH

BATHROOM TIME

	wet	b.m.
	wet	b.m.
	wet	b.m.
	wet	b.m.

SLEEP TIME

TIME	LENGTH

Snacks

MY DAY WAS

○ Good   ○ Fair   ○ Poor

Meals

Morning	○ Good	○ Fair	○ Poor
Evening	○ Good	○ Fair	○ Poor

DAILY GOALS

ACTIVITY	LENGTH	MEDICINE	TIME	DOSAGE

SEXUAL HEALTH

SYMPTOMS	RATE				
	Very Poor	Poor	Fair	Good	Excellent
	○	○	○	○	○
	○	○	○	○	○
	○	○	○	○	○
	○	○	○	○	○
	○	○	○	○	○

NOTES

Daily routine

____ / ____ / ____

M T W T F S S

OUTSIDE TIME

TIME	LENGTH

BATHROOM TIME

	wet	b.m.
	wet	b.m.
	wet	b.m.
	wet	b.m.

SLEEP TIME

TIME	LENGTH

Snacks

MY DAY WAS

○ Good   ○ Fair   ○ Poor

Meals

Morning   ○ Good   ○ Fair   ○ Poor

Evening   ○ Good   ○ Fair   ○ Poor

DAILY GOALS

ACTIVITY	LENGTH	MEDICINE	TIME	DOSAGE

SEXUAL HEALTH

SYMPTOMS	RATE				
	Very Poor	Poor	Fair	Good	Excellent
	○	○	○	○	○
	○	○	○	○	○
	○	○	○	○	○
	○	○	○	○	○
	○	○	○	○	○

NOTES

317

Daily routine

____ / ____ / ____

M	T	W	T	F	S	S
●	●	●	●	●	●	●

OUTSIDE TIME

TIME	LENGTH

BATHROOM TIME

	wet	b.m.
	wet	b.m.
	wet	b.m.
	wet	b.m.

SLEEP TIME

TIME	LENGTH

Snacks

MY DAY WAS

○ **Good**   ○ **Fair**   ○ **Poor**

Meals

Morning	○ Good	○ Fair	○ Poor
Evening	○ Good	○ Fair	○ Poor

DAILY GOALS

ACTIVITY	LENGTH	MEDICINE	TIME	DOSAGE

SEXUAL HEALTH

SYMPTOMS	Very Poor	Poor	Fair	Good	Excellent
	○	○	○	○	○
	○	○	○	○	○
	○	○	○	○	○
	○	○	○	○	○
	○	○	○	○	○

RATE

NOTES

Daily routine

____ / ____ / ____

M   T   W   T   F   S   S

OUTSIDE TIME	
TIME	LENGTH

BATHROOM TIME		
	wet	b.m.
	wet	b.m.
	wet	b.m.
	wet	b.m.

SLEEP TIME	
TIME	LENGTH

Snacks

MY DAY WAS

○ **Good**   ○ **Fair**   ○ **Poor**

Meals

Morning	○ Good	○ Fair	○ Poor
Evening	○ Good	○ Fair	○ Poor

DAILY GOALS

ACTIVITY	LENGTH	MEDICINE	TIME	DOSAGE

SEXUAL HEALTH					
SYMPTOMS	RATE				
	Very Poor	Poor	Fair	Good	Excellent
	○	○	○	○	○
	○	○	○	○	○
	○	○	○	○	○
	○	○	○	○	○
	○	○	○	○	○

NOTES

Daily routine

____ / ____ / ____

M	T	W	T	F	S	S
●	●	●	●	●	●	●

OUTSIDE TIME

TIME	LENGTH

BATHROOM TIME

	wet	b.m.
	wet	b.m.
	wet	b.m.
	wet	b.m.

SLEEP TIME

TIME	LENGTH

Snacks

MY DAY WAS

○ Good   ○ Fair   ○ Poor

Meals

Morning	○ Good	○ Fair	○ Poor
Evening	○ Good	○ Fair	○ Poor

DAILY GOALS

ACTIVITY	LENGTH	MEDICINE	TIME	DOSAGE

SEXUAL HEALTH

SYMPTOMS	RATE				
	Very Poor	Poor	Fair	Good	Excellent
	○	○	○	○	○
	○	○	○	○	○
	○	○	○	○	○
	○	○	○	○	○
	○	○	○	○	○

NOTES

Daily routine

____ / ____ / ____

	M	T	W	T	F	S	S
	●	●	●	●	●	●	●

OUTSIDE TIME

TIME	LENGTH

BATHROOM TIME

		wet	b.m.
		wet	b.m.
		wet	b.m.
		wet	b.m.

SLEEP TIME

TIME	LENGTH

Snacks

MY DAY WAS

○ **Good**   ○ **Fair**   ○ **Poor**

Meals

Morning	○ Good	○ Fair	○ Poor
Evening	○ Good	○ Fair	○ Poor

DAILY GOALS

ACTIVITY	LENGTH	MEDICINE	TIME	DOSAGE

SEXUAL HEALTH

SYMPTOMS	RATE				
	Very Poor	Poor	Fair	Good	Excellent
	○	○	○	○	○
	○	○	○	○	○
	○	○	○	○	○
	○	○	○	○	○
	○	○	○	○	○

NOTES

Daily routine

___ / ___ / ___

M	T	W	T	F	S	S
●	●	●	●	●	●	●

OUTSIDE TIME

TIME	LENGTH

BATHROOM TIME

	wet	b.m.
	wet	b.m.
	wet	b.m.
	wet	b.m.

SLEEP TIME

TIME	LENGTH

Snacks

MY DAY WAS

○ Good   ○ Fair   ○ Poor

Meals

Morning	○ Good	○ Fair	○ Poor
Evening	○ Good	○ Fair	○ Poor

DAILY GOALS

ACTIVITY	LENGTH	MEDICINE	TIME	DOSAGE

SEXUAL HEALTH

SYMPTOMS	RATE				
	Very Poor	Poor	Fair	Good	Excellent
	○	○	○	○	○
	○	○	○	○	○
	○	○	○	○	○
	○	○	○	○	○
	○	○	○	○	○

NOTES

Daily routine

___ / ___ / ___

M	T	W	T	F	S	S
●	●	●	●	●	●	●

OUTSIDE TIME

TIME	LENGTH

BATHROOM TIME

	wet	b.m.
	wet	b.m.
	wet	b.m.
	wet	b.m.

SLEEP TIME

TIME	LENGTH

Snacks

MY DAY WAS

○ **Good**   ○ **Fair**   ○ **Poor**

Meals

Morning	○ **Good**	○ **Fair**	○ **Poor**
Evening	○ **Good**	○ **Fair**	○ **Poor**

DAILY GOALS

ACTIVITY	LENGTH	MEDICINE	TIME	DOSAGE

SEXUAL HEALTH

SYMPTOMS	RATE				
	Very Poor	**Poor**	**Fair**	**Good**	**Excellent**
	○	○	○	○	○
	○	○	○	○	○
	○	○	○	○	○
	○	○	○	○	○
	○	○	○	○	○

NOTES

Daily routine

____ / ____ / ____

M	T	W	T	F	S	S
●	●	●	●	●	●	●

OUTSIDE TIME

TIME	LENGTH

BATHROOM TIME

	wet	b.m.
	wet	b.m.
	wet	b.m.
	wet	b.m.

SLEEP TIME

TIME	LENGTH

Snacks

MY DAY WAS

○ **Good**   ○ **Fair**   ○ **Poor**

Meals

Morning	○ **Good**	○ **Fair**	○ **Poor**
Evening	○ **Good**	○ **Fair**	○ **Poor**

DAILY GOALS

ACTIVITY	LENGTH	MEDICINE	TIME	DOSAGE

SEXUAL HEALTH

SYMPTOMS	RATE				
	Very Poor	Poor	Fair	Good	Excellent
	○	○	○	○	○
	○	○	○	○	○
	○	○	○	○	○
	○	○	○	○	○
	○	○	○	○	○

NOTES

Daily routine

____ / ____ / ____

M	T	W	T	F	S	S
●	●	●	●	●	●	●

OUTSIDE TIME

TIME	LENGTH

BATHROOM TIME

	wet	b.m.
	wet	b.m.
	wet	b.m.
	wet	b.m.

SLEEP TIME

TIME	LENGTH

Snacks

MY DAY WAS

○ Good   ○ Fair   ○ Poor

Meals

Morning	○ Good	○ Fair	○ Poor
Evening	○ Good	○ Fair	○ Poor

DAILY GOALS

ACTIVITY	LENGTH	MEDICINE	TIME	DOSAGE

SEXUAL HEALTH

SYMPTOMS	RATE				
	Very Poor	Poor	Fair	Good	Excellent
	○	○	○	○	○
	○	○	○	○	○
	○	○	○	○	○
	○	○	○	○	○
	○	○	○	○	○

NOTES

Daily routine

___ / ___ / ___

M	T	W	T	F	S	S
●	●	●	●	●	●	●

OUTSIDE TIME

TIME	LENGTH

BATHROOM TIME

	wet	b.m.
	wet	b.m.
	wet	b.m.
	wet	b.m.

SLEEP TIME

TIME	LENGTH

Snacks

MY DAY WAS

○ Good   ○ Fair   ○ Poor

Meals

Morning	○ Good	○ Fair	○ Poor
Evening	○ Good	○ Fair	○ Poor

DAILY GOALS

ACTIVITY	LENGTH	MEDICINE	TIME	DOSAGE

SEXUAL HEALTH

SYMPTOMS	RATE				
	Very Poor	Poor	Fair	Good	Excellent
	○	○	○	○	○
	○	○	○	○	○
	○	○	○	○	○
	○	○	○	○	○
	○	○	○	○	○

NOTES

Daily routine

___ / ___ / ___

M	T	W	T	F	S	S
•	•	•	•	•	•	•

OUTSIDE TIME

TIME	LENGTH

BATHROOM TIME

		wet	b.m.
		wet	b.m.
		wet	b.m.
		wet	b.m.

SLEEP TIME

TIME	LENGTH

Snacks

MY DAY WAS

○ **Good**   ○ **Fair**   ○ **Poor**

Meals

Morning	○ **Good**	○ **Fair**	○ **Poor**
Evening	○ **Good**	○ **Fair**	○ **Poor**

DAILY GOALS

ACTIVITY	LENGTH	MEDICINE	TIME	DOSAGE

SEXUAL HEALTH

SYMPTOMS	RATE				
	Very Poor	Poor	Fair	Good	Excellent
	○	○	○	○	○
	○	○	○	○	○
	○	○	○	○	○
	○	○	○	○	○
	○	○	○	○	○

NOTES

Daily routine

____ / ____ / ____

	M	T	W	T	F	S	S
	●	●	●	●	●	●	●

OUTSIDE TIME

TIME	LENGTH

BATHROOM TIME

	wet	b.m.
	wet	b.m.
	wet	b.m.
	wet	b.m.

SLEEP TIME

TIME	LENGTH

Snacks

MY DAY WAS

○ Good   ○ Fair   ○ Poor

Meals

Morning	○ Good	○ Fair	○ Poor
Evening	○ Good	○ Fair	○ Poor

DAILY GOALS

ACTIVITY	LENGTH	MEDICINE	TIME	DOSAGE

SEXUAL HEALTH

SYMPTOMS	RATE				
	Very Poor	Poor	Fair	Good	Excellent
	○	○	○	○	○
	○	○	○	○	○
	○	○	○	○	○
	○	○	○	○	○
	○	○	○	○	○

NOTES

Daily routine

____ / ____ / ____

M   T   W   T   F   S   S

OUTSIDE TIME

TIME	LENGTH

BATHROOM TIME

	wet	b.m.
	wet	b.m.
	wet	b.m.
	wet	b.m.

SLEEP TIME

TIME	LENGTH

Snacks

MY DAY WAS

○ Good   ○ Fair   ○ Poor

Meals

Morning	○ Good	○ Fair	○ Poor
Evening	○ Good	○ Fair	○ Poor

DAILY GOALS

ACTIVITY	LENGTH	MEDICINE	TIME	DOSAGE

SEXUAL HEALTH

SYMPTOMS	RATE				
	Very Poor	Poor	Fair	Good	Excellent
	○	○	○	○	○
	○	○	○	○	○
	○	○	○	○	○
	○	○	○	○	○
	○	○	○	○	○

NOTES

Daily routine

____ / ____ / ____

M	T	W	T	F	S	S
•	•	•	•	•	•	•

OUTSIDE TIME

TIME	LENGTH

BATHROOM TIME

	wet	b.m.
	wet	b.m.
	wet	b.m.
	wet	b.m.

SLEEP TIME

TIME	LENGTH

Snacks

MY DAY WAS

○ **Good**   ○ **Fair**   ○ **Poor**

Meals

Morning	○ **Good**	○ **Fair**	○ **Poor**
Evening	○ **Good**	○ **Fair**	○ **Poor**

DAILY GOALS

ACTIVITY	LENGTH	MEDICINE	TIME	DOSAGE

SEXUAL HEALTH

SYMPTOMS	RATE				
	Very Poor	Poor	Fair	Good	Excellent
	○	○	○	○	○
	○	○	○	○	○
	○	○	○	○	○
	○	○	○	○	○
	○	○	○	○	○

NOTES

Daily routine

____ / ____ / ____

M   T   W   T   F   S   S

OUTSIDE TIME

TIME	LENGTH

BATHROOM TIME

	wet	b.m.
	wet	b.m.
	wet	b.m.
	wet	b.m.

SLEEP TIME

TIME	LENGTH

Snacks

MY DAY WAS

○ **Good**   ○ **Fair**   ○ **Poor**

Meals

Morning   ○ **Good**   ○ **Fair**   ○ **Poor**

Evening   ○ **Good**   ○ **Fair**   ○ **Poor**

DAILY GOALS

ACTIVITY	LENGTH	MEDICINE	TIME	DOSAGE

SEXUAL HEALTH

SYMPTOMS	RATE				
	Very Poor	Poor	Fair	Good	Excellent
	○	○	○	○	○
	○	○	○	○	○
	○	○	○	○	○
	○	○	○	○	○
	○	○	○	○	○

NOTES

331

Daily routine

____ / ____ / ____

M T W T F S S

OUTSIDE TIME

TIME	LENGTH

BATHROOM TIME

	wet	b.m.
	wet	b.m.
	wet	b.m.
	wet	b.m.

SLEEP TIME

TIME	LENGTH

Snacks

MY DAY WAS

○ Good   ○ Fair   ○ Poor

Meals

Morning	○ Good	○ Fair	○ Poor
Evening	○ Good	○ Fair	○ Poor

DAILY GOALS

ACTIVITY	LENGTH	MEDICINE	TIME	DOSAGE

SEXUAL HEALTH

SYMPTOMS	RATE				
	Very Poor	Poor	Fair	Good	Excellent
	○	○	○	○	○
	○	○	○	○	○
	○	○	○	○	○
	○	○	○	○	○
	○	○	○	○	○

NOTES

Daily routine

____ / ____ / ____

M T W T F S S

OUTSIDE TIME

TIME	LENGTH

BATHROOM TIME

	wet	b.m.
	wet	b.m.
	wet	b.m.
	wet	b.m.

SLEEP TIME

TIME	LENGTH

Snacks

MY DAY WAS

○ **Good**   ○ **Fair**   ○ **Poor**

Meals

Morning	○ Good	○ Fair	○ Poor
Evening	○ Good	○ Fair	○ Poor

DAILY GOALS

ACTIVITY	LENGTH	MEDICINE	TIME	DOSAGE

SEXUAL HEALTH

SYMPTOMS	RATE				
	Very Poor	Poor	Fair	Good	Excellent
	○	○	○	○	○
	○	○	○	○	○
	○	○	○	○	○
	○	○	○	○	○
	○	○	○	○	○

NOTES

333

Daily routine

____ / ____ / ____

M	T	W	T	F	S	S
●	●	●	●	●	●	●

OUTSIDE TIME

TIME	LENGTH

BATHROOM TIME

		wet	b.m.
		wet	b.m.
		wet	b.m.
		wet	b.m.

SLEEP TIME

TIME	LENGTH

Snacks

MY DAY WAS

○ **Good**   ○ **Fair**   ○ **Poor**

Meals

Morning	○ Good	○ Fair	○ Poor
Evening	○ Good	○ Fair	○ Poor

DAILY GOALS

ACTIVITY	LENGTH	MEDICINE	TIME	DOSAGE

SEXUAL HEALTH

SYMPTOMS	RATE				
	Very Poor	Poor	Fair	Good	Excellent
	○	○	○	○	○
	○	○	○	○	○
	○	○	○	○	○
	○	○	○	○	○
	○	○	○	○	○

NOTES

Daily routine

___ / ___ / ___

M	T	W	T	F	S	S
●	●	●	●	●	●	●

OUTSIDE TIME

TIME	LENGTH

BATHROOM TIME

	wet	b.m.
	wet	b.m.
	wet	b.m.
	wet	b.m.

SLEEP TIME

TIME	LENGTH

Snacks

MY DAY WAS

○ Good   ○ Fair   ○ Poor

Meals

Morning	○ Good	○ Fair	○ Poor
Evening	○ Good	○ Fair	○ Poor

DAILY GOALS

ACTIVITY	LENGTH	MEDICINE	TIME	DOSAGE

SEXUAL HEALTH

SYMPTOMS	RATE				
	Very Poor	Poor	Fair	Good	Excellent
	○	○	○	○	○
	○	○	○	○	○
	○	○	○	○	○
	○	○	○	○	○
	○	○	○	○	○

NOTES

335

Daily routine

_____ / _____ / _____

M T W T F S S

OUTSIDE TIME

TIME	LENGTH

BATHROOM TIME

	wet	b.m.
	wet	b.m.
	wet	b.m.
	wet	b.m.

SLEEP TIME

TIME	LENGTH

Snacks

MY DAY WAS

○ Good   ○ Fair   ○ Poor

Meals

Morning	○ Good	○ Fair	○ Poor
Evening	○ Good	○ Fair	○ Poor

DAILY GOALS

ACTIVITY	LENGTH	MEDICINE	TIME	DOSAGE

SEXUAL HEALTH

SYMPTOMS	RATE				
	Very Poor	Poor	Fair	Good	Excellent
	○	○	○	○	○
	○	○	○	○	○
	○	○	○	○	○
	○	○	○	○	○
	○	○	○	○	○

NOTES

Daily routine

____ / ____ / ____

M	T	W	T	F	S	S
•	•	•	•	•	•	•

OUTSIDE TIME

TIME	LENGTH

BATHROOM TIME

	wet	b.m.
	wet	b.m.
	wet	b.m.
	wet	b.m.

SLEEP TIME

TIME	LENGTH

Snacks

MY DAY WAS

○ Good   ○ Fair   ○ Poor

Meals

| Morning | ○ Good | ○ Fair | ○ Poor |
| Evening | ○ Good | ○ Fair | ○ Poor |

DAILY GOALS

ACTIVITY	LENGTH	MEDICINE	TIME	DOSAGE

SEXUAL HEALTH

SYMPTOMS	RATE				
	Very Poor	Poor	Fair	Good	Excellent
	○	○	○	○	○
	○	○	○	○	○
	○	○	○	○	○
	○	○	○	○	○
	○	○	○	○	○

NOTES

Daily routine

____ / ____ / ____

| M | T | W | T | F | S | S |

OUTSIDE TIME

TIME	LENGTH

BATHROOM TIME

	wet	b.m.
	wet	b.m.
	wet	b.m.
	wet	b.m.

SLEEP TIME

TIME	LENGTH

Snacks

MY DAY WAS

○ Good   ○ Fair   ○ Poor

Meals

| Morning | ○ Good | ○ Fair | ○ Poor |
| Evening | ○ Good | ○ Fair | ○ Poor |

DAILY GOALS

ACTIVITY	LENGTH	MEDICINE	TIME	DOSAGE

SEXUAL HEALTH

SYMPTOMS	RATE				
	Very Poor	Poor	Fair	Good	Excellent
	○	○	○	○	○
	○	○	○	○	○
	○	○	○	○	○
	○	○	○	○	○
	○	○	○	○	○

NOTES

Daily routine

____ / ____ / ____

M	T	W	T	F	S	S
●	●	●	●	●	●	●

OUTSIDE TIME

TIME	LENGTH

BATHROOM TIME

	wet	b.m.
	wet	b.m.
	wet	b.m.
	wet	b.m.

SLEEP TIME

TIME	LENGTH

Snacks

MY DAY WAS

○ **Good**   ○ **Fair**   ○ **Poor**

Meals

Morning	○ **Good**	○ **Fair**	○ **Poor**
Evening	○ **Good**	○ **Fair**	○ **Poor**

DAILY GOALS

ACTIVITY	LENGTH	MEDICINE	TIME	DOSAGE

SEXUAL HEALTH

SYMPTOMS	RATE				
	Very Poor	Poor	Fair	Good	Excellent
	○	○	○	○	○
	○	○	○	○	○
	○	○	○	○	○
	○	○	○	○	○
	○	○	○	○	○

NOTES

_____

_____

_____

_____

_____

_____

_____

_____

_____

_____

_____

_____

_____

_____

_____

_____

_____

_____

_____

_____

_____

_____

_____

_____

_____

_____

_____

_____

_____

_____

_____

_____

_____

Notes

_____

_____

_____

_____

_____

_____

_____

_____

_____

_____

_____

_____

_____

_____

_____

_____

_____

_____

_____

Notes

Notes

Notes

Notes

_____

_____

_____

_____

_____

_____

_____

_____

_____

_____

_____

_____

_____

_____

_____

_____

_____

Notes

Notes

Notes

_____

_____

_____

_____

_____

_____

_____

_____

_____

_____

_____

_____

_____

_____

_____

Come on & Check-up on it

Notes

_____

Notes

Notes

Notes

_____

_____

_____

_____

_____

_____

_____

_____

_____

_____

_____

_____

_____

_____

_____

_____

Notes

_____

_____

_____

_____

_____

_____

_____

_____

_____

_____

_____

_____

_____

_____

_____

Notes

Notes

_____

_____

_____

_____

_____

_____

_____

_____

_____

_____

_____

_____

_____

_____

Notes

Notes

_____

_____

_____

_____

_____

_____

_____

_____

_____

_____

_____

_____

_____

_____

Come on & Check-up on it

Notes

_____

Notes

_____

_____

_____

_____

_____

_____

_____

_____

_____

_____

_____

_____

_____

_____

_____

_____

_____

_____

Notes

_____

_____

_____

_____

_____

_____

_____

_____

_____

_____

_____

_____

_____

_____

_____

_____

_____

_____

_____

Notes

_____

_____

_____

_____

_____

_____

_____

_____

_____

_____

_____

_____

_____

_____

_____

_____

_____

Notes

Notes

Notes

_____

_____

_____

_____

_____

_____

_____

_____

_____

_____

_____

_____

_____

_____

_____

_____

_____

Notes

_____

_____

_____

_____

_____

_____

_____

_____

_____

_____

_____

_____

_____

_____

_____

_____

_____

_____

_____

_____

_____

_____

_____

_____

_____

_____

_____

_____

_____

_____

_____

_____

_____

_____

Notes

_____

_____

_____

_____

_____

_____

_____

_____

_____

_____

_____

_____

_____

_____

_____

_____

_____

_____

_____

_____

Notes

_____

_____

_____

_____

_____

_____

_____

_____

_____

_____

_____

_____

_____

_____

_____

_____

Notes

_____

_____

_____

_____

_____

_____

_____

_____

_____

_____

_____

_____

_____

_____

_____

_____

Notes

_____

_____

_____

_____

_____

_____

_____

_____

_____

_____

_____

_____

_____

_____

_____

Notes

Notes

_____

_____

_____

_____

_____

_____

_____

_____

_____

_____

_____

_____

_____

_____

_____

_____

Notes

_____

_____

_____

_____

_____

_____

_____

_____

_____

_____

_____

_____

_____

_____

_____

_____

_____

Notes

Notes

_____

_____

_____

_____

_____

_____

_____

_____

_____

_____

_____

_____

_____

_____

_____

Notes

Notes

Notes

Notes

_____

_____

_____

_____

_____

_____

_____

_____

_____

_____

_____

_____

_____

_____

_____

_____

_____

_____

_____

_____

_____

_____

_____

_____

_____

_____

_____

_____

_____

_____

_____

_____

Notes

_____

_____

_____

_____

_____

_____

_____

_____

_____

_____

_____

_____

_____

_____

_____

Notes

_____

_____

_____

_____

_____

_____

_____

_____

_____

_____

_____

_____

_____

_____

_____

_____

_____

_____

_____

Notes

Notes

_____

_____

_____

_____

_____

_____

_____

_____

_____

_____

_____

_____

_____

_____

_____

Notes

Notes

Notes

_____

_____

_____

_____

_____

_____

_____

_____

_____

_____

_____

_____

_____

_____

_____

_____

_____

_____

Come on & Check-up on it

Notes

_____

_____

_____

_____

_____

_____

_____

_____

_____

_____

_____

_____

_____

_____

_____

_____

Notes

Notes

_____

_____

_____

_____

_____

_____

_____

_____

_____

_____

_____

_____

_____

_____

_____

_____

_____

_____

_____

_____

_____

_____

_____

_____

_____

_____

_____

_____

_____

_____

_____

_____

_____

_____

_____

Notes

Notes

_____

_____

_____

_____

_____

_____

_____

_____

_____

_____

_____

_____

_____

_____

_____

_____

_____

_____

_____

Come on & Check-up on it

Notes

Notes

Notes

Notes

Notes

Notes

_____

_____

_____

_____

_____

_____

_____

_____

_____

_____

_____

_____

_____

_____

_____

Notes

_____

_____

_____

_____

_____

_____

_____

_____

_____

_____

_____

_____

_____

_____

_____

_____

Me, Myself, and I

About the Author

Martrica is a born problem-solver and is driven by results. This journal is only fitting as the result from when life requested her to place close attention to health like everyone else. However, she rose to the occasion not just by consuming knowledge. She took actionable steps to aid in managing her health. She is a lover of life and laughter. She loves reading, traveling, walking, and spends her time amusing family and friends. Martrica was born, raised, and currently resides in St. Louis, MO. She is a program manager for a Fortune 500 company's retail supply chain.

Her favorite quote: *Sometimes, I feel discriminated against, but it does not make me angry. It merely astonishes me. How can any deny themselves the pleasure of my company? It's beyond me.* - Zora Neale Hurston

Life Motto: Don't complain without providing a solution.

Let's continue on the journey together through the Facebook group.

Check-up on it Breast Cancer 365 days to track your breast health.

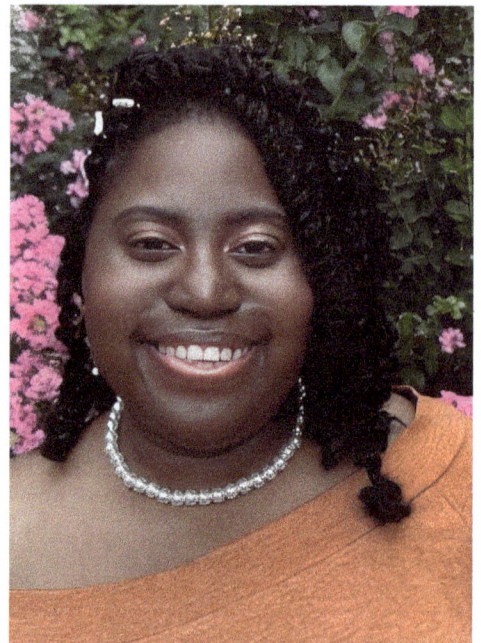

www.ingramcontent.com/pod-product-compliance
Lightning Source LLC
Chambersburg PA
CBHW080415030426

42335CB00020B/2454